Praise for *The Last Well Person*

"A brutal critique of much of what we do in medicine." *New England Journal of Medicine*

"Hadler attempts to disabuse his readers of the pervasive and arguably mistaken belief that there is good evidence to support the broad application of such things as coronary artery bypass grafting for angina; cholesterol, blood pressure, and blood glucose monitoring; and screening for colon, breast, and prostate cancer." *Canadian Medical Association Journal*

"Dr. Hadler makes a number of excellent points that are often either not discussed or underappreciated by our speciality. We need our provocateurs. We benefit from people who challenge orthodoxy and ingrained habits. Thanks to Dr. Hadler for playing that role." *Journal of Occupational and Environmental Medicine*

"I'm glad I read this book and have no hesitation in recommending it. We have a long journey ahead of us before we consistently avoid the pitfalls forthrightly identified by Hadler. Doing so will give us our best chance of having many more people remain chronically well because of rather than despite the health care system." John M Dwyer, Emeritus Professor of Medicine, Sydney, NSW, *The Medical Journal of Australia*

"So successfully has the medical industry marketed hypochondriasis that few of us escape patient-hood." Andrew Malleson, author of *Whiplash and Other Useful Illnesses*

"Any reader of *The Last Well Person* will find themselves far better off in dealing with doctors and the fluff and fine print of drug advertisements. If enough people pay attention to this book the title will be obsolete – there will be lots of well people." Anne Firor Scott, W.K. Boyd Professor of History Emerita, Duke University

"In a remarkably well-written and stimulating book Nortin M. Hadler, professor of Medicine and Microbiology/Immunology at the University of North Carolina, challenges a number of medicine's most cherished certainties. Written for the public, the book should, however, be read by all physicians and then recommended to their patients." *The Pharos*

The Last Well Person

How to Stay Well
Despite the Health-Care System

NORTIN M. HADLER, MD FACP FACR FACOEM

Professor of Medicine and Microbiology/Immunology
University of North Carolina at Chapel Hill
and Attending Rheumatologist, UNC Hospitals

McGill-Queen's University Press
Montreal & Kingston · London · Ithaca

© McGill-Queen's University Press 2004
ISBN 978-0-7735-2795-9 (cloth)
ISBN 978-0-7735-3254-0 (paper)

Legal deposit third quarter 2004
Bibliothèque nationale du Québec

Printed in Canada on acid-free paper.
Reprinted in cloth 2005
First paperback edition 2007

McGill-Queen's University Press acknowledges the support of the Canada Council for the Arts for our publishing program. We also acknowledge the financial support of the Government of Canada through the Book Publishing Industry Development Program (BPIDP) for our publishing activities.

National Library of Canada Cataloguing in Publication

Hadler, Nortin M
   The last well person: how to stay well despite the health-care system/
   Nortin M. Hadler.
   Includes bibliographical references and index.
   ISBN 978-0-7735-2795-9 (bnd)
   ISBN 978-0-7735-3254-0 (pbk)
   1. Health attitudes. 2. Health behavior. 3. Medical care – Utilization.
   I. Title.
   RA776.5.H23 2004   362.1   C2004-901742-X

Typeset in New Baskerville 11/14
by Caractéra inc., Quebec City

To a generation of students and generations of patients
for all they taught me and to
Carol S. Hadler
for making our journey together so magical

Contents

Acknowledgments

I am deeply indebted to four individuals who were willing to give generously of their time and perspective as I crafted this book. All read large sections, leaving in their wake red markings that forced me towards clarity of thinking and of prose: Clifton Meador, MD, executive director of the Vanderbilt/Meharry Alliance, who applied his finely tuned critical sense to my musings. I owe him additional kudos, since I borrowed the title of this monograph from an article he published in the *New England Journal of Medicine* in 1994. Dr Andrew Malleson, a Toronto psychiatrist, is another student of the foibles of clinical reasoning, as he well demonstrates in his monograph *Whiplash and Other Useful Illnesses*. I am profoundly grateful to Anne Firor Scott, professor emerita of history at Duke University, and Andrew Scott, professor emeritus of political science at the University of North Carolina and founder of the Coastal Carolina Press. They urged me to speak plainly and clearly, to avoid being overly self-referential, and to treat my colleagues as gently as I treat my patients. Whatever extent I succeed on any of these scores is a reflection of their efforts.

Finally, I am grateful to Rosemary Shipton, whose expert editing removed the rough edges and provided the polish.

The Last Well Person

Prologue

If you want to be well and feel well, I have written this book for you. Some of you think you are well, but occasionally you succumb to nagging doubts. Even those of you who are convinced you are well must continually withstand badgering assaults from a variety of health promoters. Some of you are overcoming encounters with illness; others are trying to put such episodes into perspective. If you really feel you are well, however, it's due to your inherent sense of invincibility. You counter any moments of uncertainty about your wellness with the firm inner conviction "I'm all right."

What, exactly, are our options as we seek to maintain this crucial sense of well-being? Life will surely threaten even those who seem most secure. We cannot live without heartache and backache, heartburn and headache, unfamiliar bowel function, peculiar sensations, days in the doldrums, realizations of physical limits, and myriad other predicaments. Each of us will experience maladies, morbid episodes that test the limits of our sense of invincibility. This book is written to bolster those personal resources that help us cope, both on our own or as we negotiate our path with professional guidance. North Americans are at a serious disadvantage on both accounts. The wealth of health information promulgated by all sorts of purveyors of health care, including the medical profession, may be intended to be helpful but often is not. Much of this information destroys our essential sense of invincibility, without doing much for either our health or our longevity. *The Last Well Person* is written for all those well people who feel their sense of well-being is under attack.

My approach is imbued with the teachings of Karl Popper and Daniel Federman. Popper moved the philosophy of science into the modern era. He placed on us all the responsibility to doubt, to question, and always to try to refute each successive "truth." Federman was one of my mentors while I was a student at Harvard Medical School and, later, a resident physician at the Massachusetts General Hospital. He remains a legend for his engaging, lucid, and comprehensive discussions as he made his rounds with his student doctors. I assumed it was a gift, but he told me later that he prepared assiduously for these seemingly extemporaneous remarks. The highest reward for any teacher is a student who learns to be insightful and questioning, and I, in turn, have spent my career as a medical educator under this banner, teaching at the bedsides of a vast array of very sick patients, both at my home institution and as visiting professor at over a hundred other places.

This practical experience forms one of the four footings on which I will build *The Last Well Person*. It is crafted to inform the reader who *is* well how to *feel* well. Rest assured, I understand the plight and circumstance of those who are not so fortunate as to be well. Otherwise, I could not appreciate the challenges to the sense of wellness that are faced by everyone who really is well.

The second footing on which I will build *The Last Well Person* is an understanding of the social consequences of illness. Thirty years ago I realized that nearly all my patients faced a plight that I had barely heard mentioned in medical school: after they left the office or the hospital, they then had to contend with the impact of the illness on their daily life and their expectations. I began to study one aspect of that plight – the need to maintain substantial gainful employment. In the years since, my interest in the "illness of work incapacity" has taken me far afield: it has forced me to explore workplaces, to analyze work and work contexts, and to probe the sociopolitical constraints imposed on both the medical community and people with disabilities as they try to connect.

An understanding of medicalization is the third footing for this book. My study of the interplay between illness and work obliged me to gain a more intimate knowledge of the perception of illness and its consequence among people who had not sought medical attention. From the physician's perspective, people who are not patients are well. However, my own work, the experience of some of my predecessors, and a vast current literature have challenged the meaning of "well" as it relates to the community at large. To be well is not to be free of symptoms, of morbidity – at least not continuously or for long. We all experience routine problems of body and mind. Sometimes we tell others, describing our plight in our own idiom of distress. Whatever we do, we are challenged to cope with these predicaments of living and life. To be well is to be able to cope with morbid episodes – and coping may not be easy. It can be thwarted by the intensity of the illness or by complicating factors such as medicalization. When the person with the problem interprets the symptoms as a medical disease, an illness for which medical treatment could or should be sought, that is medicalization. The Victorians medicalized orgasm, whereas we medicalize its lack. Medicalization superimposes a scientific idiom of distress on common sense. But common sense is not common, either temporally or geographically, and if it is sense, it's highly susceptible to presuppositions, magical thinking, and market pressures.

The fourth footing for this book is critical, rigorous science. I've already admitted to being a committed refutationist. I started my investigative career as a physical biochemist and closed my laboratory only when I found that contending with the other three footings alone was more than I could manage. However, I have a keen appreciation for the scientific method. I have applied that razor to my own epidemiological studies and to the relevant research by others. The result is a definition or even a quantification of uncertainty, not one of certainty. I am unsure about any assertion of "fact." How much uncertainty we tolerate about any fact relates to our own personal value system. Suppose I tell you that if 1,000 well people take a particular drug every day, all will be living in five years' time, whereas only 500 will survive

without the drug. Most of us would value the drug greatly, even
if its longer-term toxicities were unknown. Would you value the
drug if I told you that, after five years, there were only 510 survivors? Do you think it is possible to measure that difference
reliably? If so, do you think it is meaningful? Is it worth the
bother of swallowing the pills, the risk of short-term toxicities,
and the uncertainties in the long run? Would 550 seem more
compelling? We will revisit this scenario in chapter 1 and, repeatedly throughout the book, the topic of medical uncertainty from
the perspective of the patient.

The Last Well Person is a treatise on medicalization that is
informed by science, clinical reality, and an analysis of life's
morbid experiences – even episodes of disease. I intend to suggest ways of coping with some of the maladies that are unavoidable in the course of living as a well person. I will demonstrate
how to discern instances when medicine can offer insights in that
regard. And I will explain how to avoid iatrogenicity – medical
interventions that cause harm. Armed with scepticism and a critical intellect, it is possible to benefit, safely and effectively, from
modern medicine without being harmed in the process. It is not
my intent to speak ill of doctors, either individually or in general.
Rather, I am examining the institution of medicine, and I have
no compunctions about sharing the bad news with the good.

This book is not for people who are already seriously ill.
Coping with acute and chronic diseases that threaten your
organs, if not your life, requires a similar degree of scepticism
and a critical intellect. Although I understand the plight of those
who suffer damaging disease, I am writing here for the vast
majority – the well – who, at times, are concerned that a particular malady is more than a predicament of everyday life and fear
for their mortality.

The Last Well Person is divided into two parts. Part One tackles
the medicalization of the inevitability of death. In the academy,
this area of medical treatment is hiding under the seemingly
noble exercise of "Health Promotion, Disease Prevention" –
affectionately termed "hippie-dippie," for the acronym HPDP,
by insiders. All human beings are time bombs, we are told: we

harbour bundles of risk factors and face potential hazards that, someday, will rise up, smite us ill, and carry us off. Hippie-dippie promises to modify and mollify our mortal risks. Who can resist? Once you have read Part One, you will.

Part Two steps back from the myth of immortality to explore the medicalization of health predicaments that are normal in the course of life. If you find these chapters compelling, you will be able to confront your physician with the complaint "Doc, I feel awful. Could it be in my mind?" or "Doc, my back is killing me. I can't figure out why I can't cope with this episode." Before you read Part Two, I suspect most of you would have found the first complaint off-putting, if not infuriating, and the second, counterintuitive and difficult to do. This second half of the book is designed to change your expression of distress so it reflects your predicament rather than personal and medical presuppositions. It details how psychosocial challenges to our sense of invincibility can cause us to focus on physical and emotional symptoms in such a way that the symptoms seem more the issue than the challenges that caused us to focus in the first place. Don't read something abnormal, weak, or weak-minded into this assertion; it describes a normal dynamic. Until this explanation is grasped, however, the myriad approaches offered by others to help with the symptoms will seem seductive. Yet pursuing help for the surrogate complaint seldom provides relief, often exacerbates the symptoms, and always and forever changes that essential sense of well-being.

Teaching the well how to approach the act of medical treatment critically is something of a heresy. I am, after all, stating that neither naïveté nor trust can be counted on to serve you well. Most of the lessons I will teach are heretical as well. Without criticism and controversy, the weakness of our beliefs never surfaces. My goal is to provide you with the skills to assume responsibility for assessing your health status in the face of the barrage of information you will confront in the years to come. I am setting out to mould your critical skills so you can recognize and contend with the unfounded assertions, massaged data, and egregious marketing that have always been present but is now industrialized. There is no other way to avoid sacrificing the sense that you are well to unnecessary medicalization or, worse yet, the fact that you are well to illnesses caused by medical treatments.

Each of the ten chapters in this book is an object lesson; each tackles a topic of immediate relevance and teaches a particular skill set. I have ordered the topics so that the skills complement and build on one another. It is certainly reasonable to skip first to the chapter you find most relevant to you, and I have made some allowances in the design of the chapters for picking and choosing. However, it's best to read the book in sequence. I want to arm you to cope effectively when next you confront a personal malady or the spectre of such: to be able to consider your plight rationally, to remain in control of the choosing when there are options in recourse, and to negotiate the process with as little personal price as possible. Few are so armed. Few will be, given the climate of "health promotion." If I succeed with you, you may be the Last Well Person.

PART ONE
The Methuselah Complex

Daily we hear of the greying of America. We are offered the image of the "baby boom" generation going on forever, making impossible demands on successive generations to provide pensions, health care, and community. Forever? Fear not. The death rate is one per person. The only uncertainties in that regard are when, how it will happen, and what the journey was like.

More and more of us are living longer than did our parents. Clearly, the likelihood that we will enjoy life as an octogenarian increased over the course of the twentieth century. Far less clear is whether the prospect of our becoming a nonagenarian has similarly increased. The difference in this rate is so striking that many of us wonder if there is not a fixed longevity for our species, set around eighty-five years of age. While we can reasonably hope to live to our mid-eighties, anything beyond is a bonus and even a statistical oddity. This projected demographic is consistent with current population trends. With one caveat, these hard facts seem unlikely to change. It is possible that molecular biology can alter the fixed longevity of our species. But don't hold your breath. None of us will live to see it – and maybe no one ever will.

Part One is written with this precept in mind. I, for one, do not care how many diseases I harbour on my eighty-fifth birthday, though I prefer not to know that they are creeping up on me. Neither do I care which of these diseases carries

me off, as long as the leaving is gentle and the epilogue
meaningful. Perhaps the best we can reasonably hope for is
eighty or so years of life free of morbidities that overwhelm
our wherewithal to cope, and to die in our sleep on our
eighty-fifth birthday.

Unfortunately, not all of us will arrive at our eighty-fifth
birthday with tranquility or, having done so, have a peaceful
passing. Fortunate, indeed, are the octogenarians of today
who have the wits and faculties to contend with life's demands.
But time soon whittles away even their higher level of functional capacity. Month by month they face days when they do
not perform as usual or even feel the need to take to bed.
Inexorably, the pursuits of daily living, activities they always
took for granted, become an insurmountable challenge. They
will come to take their place among the frail elderly. They will
lean on canes by the graveside of their friends.

The hope is faint that contemporary medical science will
shepherd more of the high-functioning octogenarians into
the very meagre ranks of the high-functioning nonagenari-
ans. It is, however, possible to provide comfort and support
for these octogenarians through their transition towards
decrepitude and their final passage. Friendship, community,
and love are defensible as prescriptions and clinical interventions, and are worthy targets for public policy and expendi-
ture. To advocate otherwise, including measures purporting to
increase the lifespan beyond the mid-eighties, is to harbour
delusions of immortality. Heroic efforts on behalf of the
highly functioning octogenarians will accomplish little of
substance. We can, perhaps, alter the proximate cause of
death – the diagnosis on the death certificate – but I am
aware of no data to support the premise that we can alter the
date of death. This is not to advocate therapeutic nihilism;
rather, it is to invoke the age-old art of medicine to contend
with the reality of our aging and our mortality. When high-
functioning octogenarians decline, it is because their time is
approaching. When death supervenes, it is because it is their
time. That is the real proximate cause of death. It does not

matter how many diseases are vying for the *coup de grâce* –
only that the journey was as gratifying as possible

Although the best clinical management of frailty in
octogenarians may be support, comfort, and community,
I welcome aggressive efforts to increase the likelihood that
more members of future birth cohorts will close their lives as
highly functional octogenarians. Many people in the resource-
advantaged world still lag behind this demographic trend.
Who, in general, die before their time? Who live to a ripe
old age?

If anyone is tempted to ascribe the increasing longevity
in North America to past medical programs that promoted
health and to ongoing medical care, science tempers any
such hubris. Health-adverse behaviours and cardiovascular risk
factors may relate to the proximate cause of death, but they
account for less than 25 per cent of the hazard to longevity.
This outcome explains why multiple assaults on health-adverse
behaviours and cardiovascular risk factors have uncertain
effects on mortality rates. They might change the proximate
cause of death, but they do not alter its timing.

If we want to appreciate the good fortune of vibrant
octogenarians, we need to understand the hazards to well-
being that lurk in our ecosystem, in the world around us all.
These life-course hazards can powerfully perturb our biology
and our fate. Much of this threat can be captured by measurements of our socioeconomic status (SES). There is an
incontrovertible relationship between SES and longevity. But
do not be misled into assuming that SES is simply a measure
of income status. Longevity is more dependent on how poor
you are relative to those who are advantaged in your particular ecosystem. The greater the gap in income between the
rich and poor (the "Robin Hood index") across states in the
United States, for example, the greater the decrease in longevity of the poor. This relationship between income gap and
longevity holds across the entire advanced world. Also, do not
be misled into assuming that SES is a measure of health-care
expenditures. It isn't, not in North America or elsewhere.

SES is a measure of the kind of neighbourhood in which you live and the context in which you are employed.

A handmaiden of SES is educational status. People born between the two world wars who managed to average twelve years of education, for instance, are likely to live some seven years longer than those around them in the low SES strata. For the advantaged octogenarians, the transitions to doldrums, decrepitude, and demise are telescoped into the last year or so of life. The disadvantaged in their birth cohort commence these transitions earlier in life and suffer through their unfolding. They labour in jobs that are less rewarding, satisfying, or secure. They live under clouds of persistent pain and pervasive work incapacity. Their life is shorter and less sweet.

The great German pathologist Rudolf Virchow (1821–1902) developed a notion of "natural" as opposed to "artificial" diseases and epidemics. He considered typhus, scurvy, and tuberculosis to be "artificial" because they were primarily due to social conditions: "The artificial epidemics are attributes of society, products of a false culture, that is not distributed to all classes. They point toward deficiencies produced by the structure of the state or society, and strike therefore primarily those classes which do not enjoy the advantages of the culture."

The stratum of society that dies before its time falls victim to "artificial epidemics," which account for 75 per cent of mortal hazard. These epidemics will not respond to pharmaceuticals, nor can they be surgically excised. They play out well beyond the walls of the clinic and the hospital. They are not considered the proper target of the "Health Promotion – Disease Prevention" initiatives of contemporary medicine.

Contemporary medicine nibbles at the fray of the other 25 per cent of mortal hazard. These are the health-adverse behaviours and other biological risk factors that we hear so much about. Three chapters in Part One examine the effectiveness of this public health agenda. Clearly, this agenda is flawed from the start. For people enjoying an SES they perceive as adequate, or even advantaged, there is little to do to increase their longevity, since they are already approaching the magical eighty-five when their time is near. For the disadvantaged, those who perceive their SES as lacking, adjusting cholesterol and screening for cancer can do little to alleviate the mortal hazard of their situation in life.

EVIDENCE-BASED MEDICINE

In the five chapters in Part One, I consider topics that have occupied the careers of thousands of clinical investigators. The literature they have produced is enormous and varied. The quality of the science ranges from the overtly flawed through the anecdotal to the elegant. The intent of the science is less heterogeneous. Throughout history, clinical investigators have sought the evidence that would ground their treatments. In times past, astute observation of reproducible health effects was the only scientific method. It served well to identify such breakthroughs as colchicine for gout 2,000 years ago, vitamin B_{12} for pernicious anemia eighty years ago, and streptomycin for tuberculosis sixty years ago.

The observational method also left a paper trail and legacy of false starts, false inferences, and adverse effects of medical treatment (iatrogenicity). Tonsillectomy, for the prevention of childhood pharyngitis, is an example many older readers will recall. We learned the hard way that most children outgrew recurrent pharyngitis with or without tonsillectomy. The triumph of the last fifty years is the development of methodologies to test whether clinical inferences are valid before they are unleashed on the ill. These methodologies try to ensure that an association drawn between a stated health effect and any drug, surgical procedure, dietary change, or other intervention is genuine. Their success derives from the design of the clinical trials and the statistical methods to handle the data. Some academic disciplines are devoted to pushing back the frontier of this methodological triumph, and certain

licensing agencies, beginning with the FDA in the 1960s, now
demand evidence of safety and efficacy before pharmaceuticals can be marketed (see chapter 6).

The ethic, the methodology, and the regulations have con-
verged to create the modern clinical trials enterprise. It is an
enormous enterprise, spewing forth trials in the thousands
and data points in the millions each year. Its output threatened to overwhelm comprehensibility and effectiveness. The
result is the spawning of yet another discipline devoted to
making sense of all this output – "evidence-based medicine,"
or EBM. Around the world, groups of investigators are sifting
through all the evidence to sort the wheat from the chaff. Yes,
there is chaff. Some trials were designed less well than others
because nuances that improve design were unappreciated or
ignored, or because of execution or even faults in data analysis. Yet it's not possible simply to ignore the inadequate trials
and rely on the remaining ones for diagnosis and treatment.
What's left is often a series of results that are remarkably
inconsistent. So the investigators revisit these "more acceptable" trials and attempt to decide, or even mathematically
model, which are the least flawed and, therefore, which conclusions are least likely to be spurious. I am not belittling this
effort. It is spearheaded by the Cochrane Collaboration, a ten-
year-old multinational undertaking supported by various federal coffers. (No pharmaceutical industry moneys are
involved, though that policy is under active reconsideration.)
The collaboration has 10,000 participants divided into work-
groups according to clinical topics. It has a registry of some
300,000 studies and has already produced 1,700 evidentiary
reviews; it has 1,300 more in the pipeline and plans for 7,000
beyond that.

Reviews from the Cochrane Collaboration pertain to nearly
every topic covered in this book, and I have taken advantage
of all of them. I also discuss their limitations in many chapters and in the relevant section of the annotated readings.
The collaboration, like other EBM investigators, is committed
to methodological excellence. The working groups try to

discern whether there *is* evidence. For the clinician and the well person faced with a decision, however, that is only the first issue. If there is evidence for some health effect, the next point is whether the evidence is likely to be reliable or whether the next clinical trial will discount it. If it is likely to be reliable, is the effect meaningful and, therefore, worthwhile? Or is the effect too trivial to bother with or not worth the tradeoff in risk? This was the point of the hypothetical trial I put forward in the preface. Without this frame of reference, our values will be uninformed and our decisions, naïve.

Part One of this book provides a frame of reference for decisions that relate to mortality. Part Two provides one for decisions that relate not to mortality but to symptoms (morbidity) and other aspects of the quality of life. As we will see, it is more difficult to make rational decisions about quality of life, given the vagaries of health effects in this area.

1

Interventional Cardiology and Kindred Delusions

Terms such as myocardial infarction or heart attack, stroke or cerebral vascular accident, and atherosclerosis or hardening of the arteries are darlings of the lay medical press. Pharmaceutical and hospital marketing budgets conspire to hang coronary artery disease like a curse, an imprecation, over North America. Pills, diets, and all manner of regimens are purveyed to ensure that blood continues to flow through the coronary arteries to keep the heart attack at bay. Failing all else, there's a technological solution – modern cardiovascular surgery and interventional cardiology. The practitioners of these crafts are heroes who apply bypass grafts, angioplasties, and stents as poultices for our stricken hearts and thereby ward off the grim reaper. They are saving us from the scourge of our time, and, the message goes, we should all be poised to avail ourselves of their skill. The benefits are priceless. That's the popular image, but what's the real picture?

Coronary artery disease is no scourge – at least, no longer a scourge.

- My chance of having a heart attack at sixty is about 50 per cent less than my father's chance when he was my age.
- If my father had suffered his first heart attack when he was my age, his five-year potential for survival would have been about 50 per cent. If I have a heart attack, my likelihood of

living another five years is at least 95 per cent – without any
specific interventions.

• If I take a baby aspirin daily from the time of my first heart
  attack, the likelihood of surviving five years rises to better than
  97 per cent.

All diseases have their own histories. Bubonic plague changed
the course of the Middle Ages in Europe and then disappeared
– inexplicably – since all the elements that had supported the
pandemic were unchanged: rats, squalor, lice, the bacillus, and
so on. Rheumatoid arthritis is a twentieth-century disease, peaking in incidence and severity at mid-point. Although the pharmaceuticals in use at the time did little, if anything, to modify
its course, rheumatoid arthritis has been on the wane ever since.
Even tuberculosis had declined by the early twentieth century,
long before streptomycin, the first effective antibiotic for its
treatment, was discovered.

Myocardial infarctions and strokes are also twentieth-century
diseases. Since peaking near mid-point, their incidence has been
diminishing in all age groups. This trend started before "prevention" was said to be effective and continues despite the marginal effectiveness of public health agendas to modify "risk
factors." Of course, the diminished incidence of strokes and
even myocardial infarction is less striking in octogenarians, but
that's an issue in proximate-cause epidemiology – the exercise
that attempts to deduce which of the health hazards operating
at the time of death is most likely to have been the cause. In our
culture, everybody has to die from something, from some proximate cause, and not simply because it was "time." That's why
the decrease in the incidence of strokes, for example, is much
more striking in sixty-year-old people than in octogenarians.

There is no scientific reason for heart attacks and strokes to
hold North Americans in thrall. Yes, we all know people who
died before their time from these events, and I certainly do not
belittle the tragedy. But we know far fewer people who died
prematurely than did our parents. Aside from the socioeconom-
ically disadvantaged and those few families that are riddled with

cardiovascular problems, death before our time by myocardial infarction or stroke, although it bedevilled earlier generations, need not much concern us.

This disclaimer does not seem to make sense. We are taught that some behaviours must be avoided because they predispose us to coronary artery disease; that biochemical markers of risk must be identified and modified; and that we must be vigilant for symptoms of reduced blood supply to some part of our bodies, or pending ischemic damage, so we can avail ourselves of modern invasive cardiology and cardiovascular surgery before it is too late. I will address the "risk factors" and "health adverse behaviours" sophistry in the next chapter. Here, invasive cardiology is my focus.

ANGINA FOR SURE

Let's assume for now that our next chest pain is angina – an exercise-induced chest pain caused by inadequate blood flow to a portion of the heart muscle (the myocardium). Myocardial blood flow, or perfusion, normally increases to support the nutritional demands of exercising. Angina results when more is demanded than the blood supply to that portion can support, usually because the flow through one or more of the coronary arteries is compromised by atherosclerosis, or the build-up of fatty deposits in the blood vessels. The under-perfused portion of heart muscle is near death because of this insufficient supply of oxygen. This ischemic myocardium spews out chemicals that communicate its plight to local pain (nociceptive) nerve endings. The pain typically prevents further exercise. Without the added demand, the blood supply is adequate and the pain resolves, leaving behind a portion of the heart muscle at risk for further ischemia or even death (myocardial infarction or "heart attack").

What can be done? There are medical options, drugs that diminish the likelihood of recurrence and progression and that seem to be as effective as invasive procedures, but they are not often touted in either the lay press or, unfortunately, American clinics. If they are mentioned at all, it is usually as a trial, with the tacit, if not explicit, understanding that they are temporary. Real Americans, according to this reasoning, want to be fixed, to have the abnormality in perfusion repaired. Isn't that the triumph of modern invasive cardiology? It is only common sense, after all, and nearly every medical resident and practising physician would agree. Yet science shows that this belief system is wrong.

Sure, there has been a technological triumph. Interventional cardiologists and cardiovascular surgeons are able to alter the blood supply of the heart with a remarkably low incidence of catastrophe. But what about Type II Medical Malpractice? Type I Medical Malpractice is familiar: medical or surgical performance that is unacceptable. Type II Medical Malpractice is doing something to patients very well that was not needed in the first place – and this kind of malpractice is, at present, a scourge. Doing violence to the ischemic myocardium or its blood vessels (vasculature) is a prime example. Furthermore, if any medical procedure has no ascertainable value for the patient, there is no acceptable risk – zero. Based on compelling and robust science, interventional cardiology and cardiovascular surgery for ischemic disease stemming from atherosclerosis fit the criteria for Type II Medical Malpractice.

Atherosclerosis is a process that leads to the formation of plaques in the blood vessels. This build-up causes localized narrowing of coronary and other arteries, or, as the commonly used term describes it, "hardening of the arteries." It has a complex pathogenesis, or development process, that involves lipid deposits in the vessel lining, rapid proliferation of cells in the vessel wall, and, finally, calcification. We all are developing, if not harbouring, these atherosclerotic plaques. They are found in the coronary arteries of many young people and are ubiquitous in octogenarians. In the coronary arteries, they tend to form near the origin of the main vessels supplying the more muscular left ventricle. The narrowing can be impressive, even to the point of closure. Plaques are present in nearly everyone who has angina or has suffered a myocardial infarction – but not all. And they are present in many adults who have never experienced either one. In fact, they can occlude, or block, a coronary artery of someone who has never had either angina or myocardial infarction but who has "grown" collaterals – compensatory blood vessels branching off from other coronary arteries. Obviously, there is more to angina and myocardial infarction than the presence of plaques – and that much has been clear for decades. However, until recently the villain was said to be the plaque as it directly or indirectly blocked blood flow to the heart muscle, thereby causing angina, if not a myocardial infarction.

Today's revision of this theory is that the younger, smaller plaque is prone to develop abnormalities that allow blood clots to form. These blood clots break off and do their evil downstream, blocking blood flow to the heart muscle and causing infarction. The large, mature plaques, in contrast, develop slowly enough to allow for collaterals to compensate. This revisionist theory is responsible for a new wave of experimental pharmacology. The occluding plaque theory, however, still drives current practice.

CARDIOVASCULAR SURGERY

There are ingenious ways to diminish the effects of the occluding plaque, either by removing it or by circumventing it. Early on, several of these theories were put to the test in randomized controlled trials of intervention. Patients with angina were randomly selected to receive either the intervention designed to address the plaque directly or an intervention not so designed. One of the first trials involved pericardial poudrage – the sprinkling of a powder around the heart. The wrapping of the heart, the pericardium, is a smooth-surfaced sack. Normally, it supplements the coronary arteries as a source of nutrition and oxygen for the myocardium. This contribution is small but not trivial. The presence of a powder in the pericardial sack causes the formation of a highly vascular and granulated tissue, which, theory held, would more effectively supplement the diminished contribution of the atherosclerotic coronary arteries. In the randomized controlled trial, all the patients were anaesthetized and all underwent a skin incision, though only half received the pericardial poudrage. Yet half of both groups woke to discover that their severe angina had gone. The control patients had to have this sham surgery in order to test the effectiveness of this procedure in alleviating the symptom of angina. It turned out that the particular surgery the patients received made no difference to the outcome.

I will discuss the "placebo effect" and the ethics of sham surgery in chapter 6. It's enough to say here that a sugar pill might be an adequate control if the experiment is to test the effectiveness of another pill. And "no surgery" might be a reasonable control if the experiment is testing whether surgery alters the probability of a "hard," unequivocal, and unambiguous outcome such as death. However, there is no other way to test whether any elective surgical procedure is effective in palliating a symptom such as angina than to have a sham surgical control. A trial that compared surgery with non-surgical treatment will not suffice. I find no ethical dilemma in subjecting patients to sham surgery for this purpose. What is unethical, in my view, is to unleash any unproven elective procedures on a trusting public, treatments based only on inductive reasoning and hubris.

Following this experiment, pericardial poudrage was relegated to the archives, but not the idea of circumventing the occluding plaques. In 1959 another randomized controlled surgical trial for the treatment of angina was published. This time an artery near the heart, but not supplying the heart, was tied, or ligated, in the hope of shunting more blood to the coronary circulation. The control group again underwent a sham surgical procedure. The result of this trial was also disappointing in that nearly half the patients afforded either procedure improved. Surgery for coronary artery disease fell into disfavour – but not for long. Theory prevailed: something had to be done about circumventing plaques.

Cardiac surgery had made great strides in the repair of congenital and acquired diseases of the heart valves. Cardiac surgeons now brought the same technical competence to bear on plaques through bypass surgery – the fashioning of coronary artery bypass grafts (CABGs) to physically circumvent occluding plaques. A burgeoning specialty came into being, but not without its critics. In response to these criticisms, three large multi-centre randomized controlled trials of CABG surgery were undertaken in the late 1970s. Hundreds of patients with stable angina were recruited and randomly divided into two groups. One group had CABG surgery and the other, because sham surgery was not considered appropriate or ethical, received the optimal medical therapy of the day. Patients in one of these trials were followed for five years, and those in the other two for over a decade. The results were reported in the mid-1980s. The primary outcome studied was death.

For 97 per cent of the CABG patients in all three trials, there was no survival benefit from the surgery. A subset in all three trials, a small group with a particularly noxious distribution of plaques prominently involving the left main coronary artery (left main disease), experienced some benefit. The five-year survival rate for patients with stable angina and left main disease was 65 per cent on medical therapy, and 85 per cent if they underwent CABGs. So CABGs can provide a survival advantage – save a life – for a small subset at high risk of death. For nearly everyone else, 97 per cent of patients with angina, there is no discernible survival advantage. Medical therapy has advanced significantly in the past fifteen years, so the "control" group would do even better today. There is no data to suggest, however, that CABG surgery is more effective today than it was fifteen years ago.

In the 1970s the US Veterans Administration also carried out a multi-centre randomized controlled trial of CABG surgery for "crescendo angina" – one of several labels that denote angina so severe it occurs even without exertion; it was thought to bode evil in terms of both impending myocardial infarction and death. Yet in the VA trial, the two-month incidence of death was 2 per cent, and the five-year incidence less than 10 per cent – and that was true whether or not the patient had been subjected to a CABG.

CABGs should have been relegated to the archives fifteen years ago, but they have not. In fact, some 500,000 are still done annually in the United States. This incidence far outstrips that in all other "advanced" countries. The cardiovascular surgery community continues to announce the demonstrated 20 per cent survival benefit, but seldom the fact that the benefit pertains only to the 3 per cent of all comers with the special left main blockages. The cardiovascular surgery community speaks of benefit to patients who have multiple blockages in multiple vessels, but the basis for that claim is marginal. It derives from a reanalysis of the data from the classic trials mentioned above, a "secondary analysis" that is an indefensible statistical manoeuvre. James Mills referred to such revision in 1993 as "data torturing" and explained: "If you torture your data long enough, they will tell you whatever you want to hear." Yet this secondary analysis provides justification for all multiple bypasses. It is the fountainhead for that peculiarly American narrative of illness in which survivors of CABGs and their families speak with reverence, if not pride, of the number of grafts they received.

The surgical community does little to forewarn us of the demonstrated downside of these procedures: the anguish of the cardiac catheterizations required before surgery; the challenges of healing and recovery; the 2–8 per cent who die on the table or in the post-operative period; the 50 per cent who suffer emotional distress, mainly depression, in the first six months; the 40 per cent who have memory loss at a year; and the alarming number (depending on their level of activity before the CABG) who never return to the workforce or describe themselves again as well and enjoying life. For some, dementia is the only clinically important result of having their coronary artery anatomy successfully rearranged. For none is the likelihood of survival improved.

In reply to such criticism, the cardiovascular surgical community holds that the CABG technique has been refined since the old trials. Patients are doing so well, surgeons claim, that there is no need to repeat the three now-dated classic trials that compare surgery with medical therapy. It is argued that experience and consensus bear out the theory that bypassing plaques with the latest techniques supersedes that science. Today, the primary hypothesis relates to which procedure is best, not whether any of them really works. A colleague of mine, a prominent and respected senior cardiovascular surgeon renowned for technical prowess, put it to me this way: "If you were to hold a diseased grey heart in your hand and watch it turn pink when you established full flow through a graft, you wouldn't question the benefit of CABG." Clearly, he felt triumphant, but did his experience translate into any meaningful outcome for the patient? The data relating to in-hospital mortality and cognitive deficits pertain to recent experience, not just the early days. If these procedures were pharmaceuticals, the Food and Drug Administration would not have permitted their sale. Unfortunately, the regulation of procedures is far less stringent than the regulation of pharmaceuticals.

To minimize the risk of being fooled, researchers must define their outcomes before they begin their study. In the three classic studies noted above, the primary outcome is unequivocal: death is death. Nearly all studies since have used a "combined outcome" – usually death, myocardial infarction, or "need" for CABGs, as defined by the treating cardiologists and cardiovascular surgeons. In all these subsequent studies, whether of surgery or interventional cardiology, the interventions do not alter the likelihood of death. They may alter the likelihood of non-fatal myocardial infarction, but that is an inconsistent result. They often alter the decision whether the patient should undergo a first or a repeat CABG. However, the decision to have surgery for angina is primarily a subjective exercise, depending on the prejudice of the investigator and the gullibility of the subject. "Combined outcome" studies, then, always demand scrutiny. Whenever the outcome is subjective, as for angina or the decision to have surgery, the study must be designed so as to minimize the likelihood of biasing the result. For example, when the control group undergoes a sham procedure, the control patients' expectations as to outcome are more similar to those of the test group than if they were "just" offered a pill.

INTERVENTIONAL CARDIOLOGY

The cardiovascular surgery community has two powerful allies: it is supported by an enormously profitable, co-dependent interventional cardiology industry and by a lay press that applauds technology for technology's sake. As a result, an untenable clinical hypothesis has become a social construction. It is commonly believed, by physicians and the laity alike, that if a patient has angina, any supposedly offending plaques must be circumvented.

The need to find and banish occluding plaques has been elevated to an unalienable right for Americans who are suffering, or might be suffering, from angina. In the 1980s, American cardiology had no higher calling. How could so many cardiologists have been deluding themselves and their patients? Cardiology did take the lead in trying to spare patients the rigours of cardiovascular surgery, but not by questioning its premise. Interventional cardiologists have perfected the skill to thread all kinds of tubes through our arteries or veins, while the biotechnology industry has created a variety of devices to enhance the catheters that dismantle the offending plaques. First, in a process called angioplasty, researchers invented special catheters with balloon tips, so the tip can be inserted into the narrows of the vessel and inflated to break the plaque asunder. Many a cleared vessel became blocked again, starting, usually, with a blood clot. The outcome for the patient was much the same, whether the vessel remained unobstructed (patent) or not.

Whatever happens, interventional cardiologists strive to maintain the patency of vessels whose plaques they have attacked. Since the 1990s, the cardiology community has recommended another approach to increasing the perfusion of partially occluded coronary arteries, one practitioners regard as a modification of the cardiac catheterization procedure. They leave behind a stent, or piece of tubing, designed to keep the vessel open. And they have recruited all sorts of pharmaceutical inventiveness to that end, most designed to inhibit blood clots from forming at the site of that foreign body, the stent. The number of angioplasties in the United States each year is well over 500,000, exceeding even the number of CABGS – and many an unsuspecting patient has been afforded both. The explicit understanding between cardiologist and patient is that angioplasty and stenting are "less invasive" (though not less expensive), but, should the outcome be unfavourable,

CABG is the fallback. And if the CABG "fails," another CABG is the fallback.

The systematic trials found CABGs to be no more effective than medical therapy in improving the likelihood that a patient will live to be eighty-five years of age. I believe that the symptoms and mortality from CABGs suffered by the 97 per cent who gain no survival advantage overwhelm the 20 per cent improvement in survival among the 3 per cent with left main disease. As for angioplasties, interventional cardiology is convinced it is on the right track and sees no need for similar trials using "medical treatment" as the control. True, there have been many trials, but they test whether a particular form of angioplasty offers an advantage over another form or over CABGs. The several that compare CABGs with angioplasty generally discern no important clinical difference, so angioplasty is said to be as good as CABGs and gentler. In my interpretation, angioplasty is as bad as CABGs, even though it is significantly gentler. There are also many trials comparing one form of angioplasty with another, and others probing whether the timing of angioplasty matters – whether close to a clinical event or not. As discussed above, there are small differences, usually apparent in the "need" to go on to CABG or in the incidence of myocardial infarction, but not in survival. All this micro research is missing the big picture: there is something basically wrong with the theory that calls for violence to the offending, occluding plaque.

To abandon the theory would be to shut down interventional cardiology, nearly all of cardiovascular surgery, and many surgical supply houses and biotechnology firms. It would dramatically downsize most hospitals and critical-care units in the United States and free up over $100 billion annually. Since 1987, cardiovascular disease has been the largest source of health-care spending in the country and the costs keep escalating, with cardiologists and cardiovascular surgeons providing fodder for an enormous supporting industry. Indeed, terms such as "throughput" and "units of care" are commonly used to describe the management of patients with coronary artery disease in American health centres and hospitals.

Compared with the United States, the national health insurance schemes of other advanced countries cost a quarter of what Americans spend on the insured, have a third or less of overhead expenses, and eschew much of the Type II Medical Malpractice I decry in several chapters in this book. Yet survival statistics in all advanced countries exceed those in the United States, and their citizenry enjoys more years of high-quality life. There is also a serious problem with conflict of interest, as many cardiologists and cardiovascular surgeons have financial ties to providers of technological and pharmaceutical supplies. It's disconcerting to find that trials funded by for-profit organizations are more likely to be interpreted as positive than comparable trials funded by not-for-profit organizations. We have, indeed, a cardiovascular industry.

Evaluations, cardiac catheterization, surgical teams, hospitalization, and drugs are just the direct costs. There are also "indirect" costs that relate to income substitution and lost productivity, not to mention the personal costs of becoming a "cardiac patient" or even a "cardiac cripple." The former is the fate of all; the latter the fate of too many who are hidden from popular view. We are regaled by the legends of public figures, politicians, and football coaches who rebounded from CABGs or angioplasties as if nothing had transpired. They are the exception. Within a month of undergoing a CABG, 19 per cent of patients are readmitted to hospital because of complications. As I will explain in chapter 9, if you had no job autonomy before sliding down this cardiovascular algorithm, you will likely end up on someone's disability role.

If CABGs and angioplasty don't save lives, do they improve symptoms and reduce angina? There is little scientific data addressing this issue. An enormous trial is under way, still unpublished, comparing modern medical therapy with angioplasty. However, if we bring an open mind to the published experiences with CABGs and angioplasty, we can tentatively presuppose the results of the trial. First, in the sham surgery trials, half the subjects experienced symptomatic relief, whether in the sham or the effective group. That same result holds for thousands of placebo-controlled randomized trials of pharmaceuticals for angina. For the agents that pass regulatory muster, the effectiveness was slightly more than the 50 per cent response rate found in the placebo group. Does that mean that angina is "in your mind"? Some of the explanation relates to the natural history of angina; it is an intermittent and remittent symptom complex – meaning it can go away, even though the plaques do not. Maybe that improvement relates to the formation of collateral vessels. But perhaps, too, some of the explanation is psychological in origin. Maybe participating in a trial where there is a chance that patients will get some benefit helps them deal with the anticipation of pain more effectively or allows them to circumvent angina by subtle alterations in behaviour. For me for the time being, "in your mind" is reasonable enough as an explanation.

However, in the clinical setting, rather than the clinical trial setting, the relevant "mind" is not just the patient's; it's the treating physician's as well. Medical therapy of a symptom such as angina is not simply the prescription of a pharmaceutical. It is a treatment act of far greater dimension. The attitude of the physician will colour the attitude of the patient and prejudice the effectiveness of the treatment. We have compelling data to that effect in rheumatology, in the treatment of painful joints. If the attitude the physician projects emphasizes concerns about toxicities or ineffectiveness, the patient is less likely to be on the prescribed agent for long. In cardiology circles, the prejudice is so strong towards invasive procedures that few patients can suffer angina without receiving some form of putatively beneficial violence or even receiving it again. Both the patient's and the doctor's prejudice favours the invasive procedures, so few patients can countenance the likelihood that all were in vain. For the patient, interventional cardiology and cardiovascular surgery for coronary artery disease become truth.

STROKE

The most cerebral of subspecialties, neurology, has also countenanced some interventionalist inroads. The parallels with interventional cardiology and cardiovascular surgery are obvious: the invasive neuroradiologists are manning the catheters, and the neurosurgeons are bypassing the plaques. The parallel with angina is called a "transient ischemic attack," or TIA, in which highly disconcerting neurological deficits develop and then totally reverse within twenty-four hours. How do we know they will disappear? If they don't, the patient will have suffered a stroke (a "brain attack," to emphasize the parallels with heart attacks). People with TIAs all have plaques in the four major vessels that course through the neck to feed the brain. The plaques in the internal carotid arteries are amenable to surgery – a delicate stenting procedure that can be completed by highly experienced surgeons without too many catastrophes. Is the patient better off for the effort? A large, randomized controlled trial offered the answer, though only a part seems to have made it into the public eye. If you have TIAs *and* a very tightly occluded internal carotid artery feeding the side of the brain that is transiently ischemic, surgery will afford you a meaningful reduction in your risk of suffering a stroke on that side – meaningful enough to justify the surgical risks. But that surgery will not improve your longevity: you are likely to die at the same time, often of a stroke on the other side or of cardiac disease. Maybe the quality of your life will benefit if you are spared the stroke on the same side as the surgery, but that's only a possibility.

Another trial has excited interventional neuroradiologists and caused hospitals across the United States to staff "stroke units" in the same way they have "coronary care units." When patients develop a focal neurological deficit from an occlusion caused by a blood clot, and then, within three hours, undergo a cerebral angiogram (similar to a cardiac catheterization, but of the brain's vessels), their chances of a complete recovery are improved if drugs are infused directly into the blocked cerebral artery to dissolve the clot. That assumes they are not among the 6 per cent in whom the infusion causes far more catastrophic bleeding into the brain than nearly all strokes do. Alternatively, they could take their chances that the deficit will turn out to be a TIA, in which case taking aspirin will decrease the likelihood of recurrence, though not of stroke. And if a stroke is their fate, it is not as likely to be as catastrophic as the strokes that complicate the procedure designed to dissolve the clot.

HOW TO PREPARE

Coronary artery disease is no longer a scourge, then, and interventional cardiology and cardiovascular surgery are no solution. However, angina is an awful experience, and people do die from a myocardial infarction with or without symptoms of angina. Given the state of the science and the unconscionable record of American cardiology and cardiovascular surgery, what is a well person to do?

First, we must find a primary care physician who feels compelled to keep our welfare at the centre of treatment. It is easy to find physicians with that ethic, but nearly impossible to name one who can serve the ethic well any more. All their perspective and wisdom is squelched by a "health-care delivery system" that denigrates spending time with a patient. The us health-care system will pay our primary care physician the same whether we are expeditiously referred on to a cardiologist for symptoms of angina or treated to a discourse on the choices available. The health-care system does not support a lengthy discussion between a well person and a physician aimed at defining contingencies before the onset of angina or a myocardial infarction.

If, as individuals, we identify such a physician, we should seek to define our preferred form of treatment when we are well. This planning will not take place during an "annual physical examination," which is entirely useless. Rather, we should discuss codicils to our living will that pertain to events that fall far short of a catastrophe. For one, we might explain that, should we end up in an emergency room with chest pain from myocardial ischemia, with or without a completed infarction, we want nothing done to our heart, unless the procedure is supported by compelling scientific data as to meaningful beneficial outcomes. If the physician is not comfortable with the relevant literature, ask for a referral to some physician who is. The only way we can know our own mind in this regard is to consider options when we are well and able to consider why someone's best advice is best for us. Today, for me, that means no angioplasties, stents, or CABGs. Since I have no interest in such, there is never a reason to "define my coronary anatomy" with a cardiac catheterization study.

Once we have an expanded living will, we can safely approach the medical establishment with a complaint of chest pain, knowing our sage physician will stand between Type II Medical Malpractice and us. If the pain is awful, meet this physician in the emergency room. The standard management of an acute myocardial infarction in the United States, as with angina, veers towards Type II Medical Malpractice. However, if you have a myocardial infarction, you are no longer a candidate to be the Last Well Person – and you fall beyond the boundaries for this book. So, let's take the case of less severe chest pain. We should not hesitate to approach our wise physician with such a complaint. Describe the pain. Explain that it is too severe, or atypical, or pervasive for us to cope with on our own. We are seeking insight, free of the pressure to find a supposedly offending occlusive plaque. If it's angina, we want the best of modern medical therapy – including pharmaceuticals with some small but important effect on the frequency and intensity of episodes; pharmaceuticals, such as baby aspirin, that decrease the likelihood of suffering an infarction before we have time to form collaterals; and perhaps other agents that interfere with the pathogenesis of coronary artery disease, including agents that work on lipids. I'll have more to say about that in the next chapter. But how do we know if the chest pain is angina?

Classically, angina is a severe squeezing pain behind the breastbone that is precipitated by exercise and relieved by rest. It is described as so pervasive that few can do anything but stop all exertion. The pain has a tendency to radiate into the left arm, even as far as the base of the thumb. If sufferers place nitroglycerine under their tongue during an attack, they will promptly substitute a headache for the chest pain. If you have symptoms of this nature, it is nearly certain you have angina.

Variations in this story may still be angina. The cardiology community is committed to developing a test that makes the diagnosis of angina when the symptoms are atypical. This effort is driven by the belief that the diagnosis of angina is critical, since it leads to all the procedures I decry above. I, obviously, see no pressing need to make the diagnosis of angina. Furthermore, all the steps in the test – from exercising while monitoring the electrocardiogram (EKG) to exercise tests that more directly monitor the perfusion of the heart muscle – are not sufficient either to make a diagnosis of angina or to exclude it either. They are all bedevilled with false negatives and false positives, not to mention being expensive and anxiety provoking.

So, what should we do if the chest pain may or may not be angina? We must negotiate with our physician a clinically meaningful approach to the differential diagnosis of chest pain. There are entities that can be defined, some of which we want to know about because something can be done that advantages us in an important way. Some are tumours, some lung diseases, some other vascular diseases, while some afflict our esophagus or stomach. As long as the diagnostic exercise is defined and delineated up front and holds promise for a meaningful outcome, we should go along with it. Otherwise, why bother? Let's take our chances on natural history, get on with our lives, and trust our physician to do the worrying.

I realize that my approach countenances both uncertainty and watchful waiting in an era that denigrates both. I am no Luddite. I favour any and all diagnostic and technological advances that have been shown clearly and unequivocally to benefit the patient. Interventional cardiology and cardiovascular surgery are short on both. The Whitehall II prospective cohort study has been following British civil servants for decades, for instance, leading to many observations that are relevant here and in other chapters as well. In one analysis, a cohort of some 10,000, aged thirty-five to fifty-five at inception, were followed for eleven years. They were surveyed on five occasions between 1985 and 1999 for numerous health-related issues, including symptoms of angina, and were subjected to three electrocardiograms. Over this period, some 1,200 (11%) developed angina according to a questionnaire, but 74 per cent had no evidence of a diagnosis at the time of presentation, and most of this group remained undiagnosed, despite recurrent symptoms of angina or even the development of electrocardiographic abnormalities indicating damage to the heart muscle. The civil servants with angina but without EKG evidence of damage lived as long as those who never suffered angina, though they were more likely to be ill over time. The civil servants with angina and heart damage lived less long. But it mattered not whether the angina was diagnosed and, presumably, treated. Angina is not trivial either as an experience or as a mortal hazard. Modern medicine, however, is no match for the latter.

2

Fats, Fads, and Fate

There is no question that "cholesterol" is a "risk factor" and that the "statin" family of drugs can lower cholesterol. There is no question that lowering cholesterol in patients who have already suffered a heart attack, or myocardial infarction, will result in a small though measurable decrease in their likelihood of suffering another one, and a smaller, barely measurable increase in their survival rate. However, there are serious questions whether statin treatment affords any meaningful advantage to people who have not had a heart attack. Can we recruit science to answer those questions or even assuage the doubt?

In one multi-centre study conducted by a consortium of investigators, the West of Scotland Coronary Prevention Study Group, a program was set up to screen the blood cholesterol of healthy men aged forty-five to sixty-four. Of those with high cholesterol, 6,595 agreed to participate in a five-year randomized placebo controlled trial of pravastatin, the statin marketed under the brand name Pravachol by the sponsor for the trial, the Bristol-Myers Squibb Pharmaceutical Company. Every morning for five years, these men took a pill. For 3,302 men, that pill contained 40 mg of pravastatin; for the remainder, the pill contained a pharmacologically inert substance, a placebo. The results of this study elevated statins to the forefront in considerations of public health policy and even in recommendations by advisory panels of such organizations as the American Heart Association. We must decide if this science compels us, the well people, towards

Table 2.1
The West of Scotland Pravastatin Study

Outcomes over Five Years	Placebo (3,293 men)	Pravastatin (3,302 men)
Non-fatal heart attack	204 (6.5%)	143 (4.6%)
Death by heart attack	52 (1.7)	38 (1.2)
Death by cancer	49 (1.5)	44 (1.3)
Non-cardiovascular death	62 (1.9)	56 (1.7)
Death by any cause	135 (4.1)	106 (3.2)

cholesterol screening and, if our cholesterol level is said to be "high," towards treatment. Table 2.1 sets out the results.

Let's examine the table from the bottom up. Pravachol (in high dose) saved no lives; the difference between the numbers who died from any cause is neither statistically nor clinically meaningful. There was also no difference in the likelihood of death from non-cardiovascular causes. That's important for two reasons: deaths from stroke were not avoided, and violent deaths did not increase. The latter was a finding in several earlier studies of the effect of other cholesterol-lowering drugs. Pravachol did not increase cancer deaths, nor did it protect people from heart attacks. The difference between the percentage of men in the study who suffered a fatal myocardial infarction on placebo and on Pravachol is 1.7 per cent − 1.2 per cent = 0.5 per cent. That difference is neither statistically significant nor clinically meaningful. When the investigators shifted ten deaths out of the "non-cardiovascular" category into the "heart attack" category, because these men might have died from a heart attack, the difference was 1.9 − 1.3 = 0.6 per cent. That difference is barely statistically significant; it would happen by chance 4.2 times in 100, slightly less than the consensus cut-off for statistical significance of 5 times in 100.* On that basis, the authors of the article published in the *New England Journal of Medicine* concluded that pravastatin

---

*These cut-offs are arbitrary; it depends on how much you are willing to gamble that an infrequent event is too infrequent to occur by chance alone. I muse that winning a state lottery is too infrequent an event to occur by chance alone; there must be some unknown force.

saved lives. To my eye they are massaging the data beyond the reasonable. Even granting them their secondary analysis, a difference of 0.6 per cent is not clinically meaningful. There is simply too much "noise" in any clinical trial to be confident of such small differences – factors including flaws in design, execution, or analysis of the trial, some of which may reflect prejudice on the part of the investigators or even malfeasance. Even the most elegant of trials can fall victim to "randomization errors." Bear with me through this explanation. It is a crucial concept and necessary for the Last Well Person to be a match for all the seductive marketing schemes based on trials yielding small differences in outcomes.

The principle behind a randomized controlled drug trial is that the comparison groups are comparable in every way except for the exposure to the drug being studied. Some of the comparability can be assured by design: gender, age, and even socioeconomic status can be matched as subjects are assigned to study groups. If an even distribution of measured attributes is not assured in the process of assignment to groups, any detected discordances can be compensated for in the design of the statistical analysis of the data. So, if measurable and measured health-adverse behaviours or other known risk factors (age, for example) happen to be assigned discordantly, statistical modelling can compensate for their influence on the outcomes of the study groups. However, some crucial attributes cannot be measured. Some remain hidden because they are not yet defined (for example, genetic factors that determine collateral vessel growth and the likelihood of healing a myocardial infarct) or because measurement is not feasible. For example, researchers might like to match the groups for coronary artery anatomy so that as many individuals with severe, but asymptomatic, atherosclerosis end up in the pravastatin as in the placebo groups. However, that would entail exposing over 6,000 well men to the hazards of a cardiac catheterization. The researchers proceed on the assumption that the random assignment of the men will equalize these unmeasured confounders, or variables. But what if it doesn't? What if, instead of 50–50, those with severe subclinical atherosclerosis distribute 49–51, or 48–52? Since the disparity is unmeasured, it can well account for the o.6 per cent difference in outcome. For that reason, I discount as unbelievable any statistically significant result that represents a tiny outcome. My cut-off for credibility starts at 2 per cent and approaches my comfort level at 5 per cent – and that pertains to the difference in a clinically meaningful "hard" outcome such as death or a definite non-fatal myocardial infarction. (For a soft outcome such as angina or "need" for coronary artery bypass grafts, I am not comfortable till the difference between intervention and control approaches 20 per cent.) There are others who are even more stringent. Yet this uncertainty does not seem to trouble many who design and analyze drug trials, or those who trumpet the results.

Is 2 per cent clinically meaningful? Is it meaningful to you? In table 2.1, 2 per cent reduction in non-fatal heart attacks over five years is what we're being offered as the statistically significant finding, likely to occur by chance fewer than one time in 1,000. If a well man with high cholesterol takes 40 mg of Pravachol every day, his risk of a non-fatal myocardial infarction over the course of five years is reduced nearly 2 per cent: 6.5 per cent – 4.6 per cent = 1.9 per cent. Again, I ask, is this important to you? In the published study of the trial and in subsequent marketing, the purveyors of Pravachol seldom describe the result as a 1.9 per cent reduction in the likelihood of suffering a non-fatal heart attack in five years – which is the reduction in *absolute* risk. They are wont to talk about the reduction in *relative* risk – which is the percentage that the risk for the men on placebo would be reduced if they were to swallow Pravachol: 1.9/6.5 = 0.29, or 29 per cent. In other words, they were 29 per cent less likely to suffer a non-fatal heart attack if they took Pravachol. That's true, and it certainly seems impressive. But the absolute reduction in likelihood is what is meaningful to the population at large – and that's 2 per cent. Talk of relative risk reduction without a statement of absolute risk reduction is meaningless. The real question is whether this 2 per cent reduction in absolute risk of not suffering a non-fatal heart attack in five years is worth taking Pravachol every morning.

- In chapter 1, I said that my likelihood of surviving for five years after my first heart attack was about 95 per cent. If I take a daily baby aspirin, the likelihood rises to about 97.5 per cent. That's a 2.5 per cent absolute risk reduction. (It's half of my total risk of 5 per cent, so it's a 50 per cent relative risk reduction.) The many studies of the hazards of long-term low-dose aspirin therapy show that there may be a very small increase in the likelihood of intestinal bleeding, but the hazard is overwhelmed by the 2.5 per cent reduction in the absolute risk of death after a first heart attack. If you have had a heart attack, it makes sense to take a baby aspirin daily for the rest of your life. But should you, as a well person who has never had a heart attack or a gastrointestinal bleeding episode, decide to take a baby aspirin every day as a precaution against having your first attack? The absolute risk reduction for the primary prevention of a heart attack, if there's any risk reduction at all, is minuscule. The absolute risk of intestinal bleeding from taking a baby aspirin every day is also minuscule. It's your call.
- What about statins? What is the personal benefit/risk assessment for a statin? Does the 1.9 per cent reduction in risk of a non-fatal heart attack advantage a well person with high blood cholesterol enough to justify taking Pravachol forever? Many elements enter into such an assessment. Cost may be one issue, particularly for the "health-care delivery system." The costs of a screening program and the treatment of 7 per cent or more of males between the ages of forty-five and sixty-four are substantial. The pharmaco-economists leap to that challenge. They typically focus on the 0.6 per cent absolute reduction in the risk for death from definite/possible heart attacks – the 0.6 per cent I dismissed as unreliable. If you accept the 0.6 per cent as valid, you can calculate the number

of people you need to treat (the "number needed to treat," or NNT) for five years to save one life. The result of such NNT calculations based on the West of Scotland study is generally in the 200 range.* You can also calculate the number of lives you will save in five years for the cost of having all the well men swallow Pravacol. Generally, if the calculation comes out less than US$50,000 per year of life saved, the drug is deemed worthy and the purveyor gains an edge with the Food and Drug Administration, with managed care and other insurers, Medicare and Medicaid, prescribing physicians, and the public. A cost per life-year gained for primary prevention with pravastatin in the United Kingdom was calculated to be $34,640 in 1997. If, as I suspect, Pravachol saves no lives, we are all paying a great deal of money for nothing. In fact, we may be paying a great deal of money for worse than nothing.

• If cost is not a personal issue, probably because of drug insurance plans, are there other personal risks to taking Pravachol that might mollify the 1.9 per cent reduction in the risk of a non-fatal heart attack? Some people get a rash, or headache, or some nausea, but then they can opt to stop the therapy. Statins can cause a severe, even deadly destruction of muscles. That's rare, but the benefits are too slight to tolerate much risk. One statin, Baycol, was pulled from the market because of fifty or more cases of fatal myositis. Fewer such catastrophes have been reported for the other statins, but some have been reported with exposure to each of the statins along with a number of cases with milder and reversible

---

*Of course, this calculation depends on which outcome you choose to treat for. If you assume you can effectively treat to prevent both fatal and non-fatal heart attacks, the NNT per year with Pravachol has been calculated at 217 to save one life – a result similar to another study treating well people with a different statin. The calculations for treating ill people with established coronary heart disease vary between 63 and 167.

muscle toxicity.* There's the rub. I can't tell you the long-term risk of statins; they are a unique class of agents and our long-term experience is limited. For all I know, insidiously progressive muscle disease, liver disease, or cognitive impairment lurks in the distant future of some of the men who have yielded to the persuasion that a 1.9 per cent absolute risk reduction in non-fatal myocardial infarction over the course of the next five years is valuable. Some may come to regret that the "standard of care" practised by their physician and the direct-to-consumer marketing on television by a former football coach were allowed to colour their sense that they were well.

Ten per cent of all drugs approved for marketing by the FDA between 1975 and 1999 were subsequently either withdrawn from the market because of adverse reactions or labelled with a "black box" indicating special hazards. There is much to be said for avoiding the use of any new drug unless there is compelling data that it offers an important benefit that does not derive from older agents. I do not allow "samples" in my clinic and do not allow pharmaceutical "detail" people to try to convince me that the agent they market is indispensable. I do not want to be swayed by the convenience of samples nor do I wish to delegate benefit/risk assessments. I assume responsibility

---

*Post-marketing monitoring for drug toxicity after regulatory approval – called Phase IV drug trials – is neither systematic nor comprehensive in the short or long term. It is seldom pursued unless driven by a product liability lawsuit. The FDA relies, instead, on Phase III randomized controlled trials. They often recruit thousands of subjects, seek the statistical power to detect small difference in effectiveness, and last a year or so. Post-licensing, the agent can be prescribed to tens of thousands for many years. As with Baychol, it takes the appearance of only fifty tragedies from unique complications to spot the toxicity and assign its cause. However, a marked increase in the occurrence of a disease with a significant background incidence – dementia, for example – will be missed if we rely solely on a haphazard reporting mechanism.

for assessing the available clinical trials as to efficacy of the touted drug. And I wait several years before I prescribe any new agent with equivocal benefit. I want the empirical, inefficient post-marketing surveillance system to offer some reassurance that prescribing any supposedly more effective or more convenient agent has no dire consequences.

• Even if my uneasiness about the long-term toxicity of statins turns out to be unfounded, there remains the risk of "negative labelling." We have known for twenty years that many people feel stigmatized once they are diagnosed as hypercholesterolemic. Once labelled, they feel vulnerable. Their coping skills are challenged, and they can rapidly disappear from the ranks of the well forever. The same consequence of labelling has been shown for the "hypertension," "sickle trait," and several other diagnoses.

Other statins have been tested for effectiveness in primary prevention. One was a trial of lovostatin in well US Air Force personnel with normal blood cholesterol. However, none of these trials offers more compelling support for a "public health" agenda to pharmacologically lower the blood cholesterol of well people than the West of Scotland Study. Most other studies are negative; a few suggest harm. The Air Force prophylactic statin study has results consonant with, but no more compelling than, the West of Scotland Study in demonstrating the slight efficacy of lovostatin. To further muddy the waters, the West of Scotland Study result did not reproduce in a randomized controlled trial in the United States, the "Antihypertensive and Lipid-Lowering Treatment to Prevent Heart Attack Trial" (ALLHAT-LLT). Over 10,000 men and women, aged fifty-five or older, were randomized to receive pravastatin or "usual care" in a trial conducted in some 500 different clinics around the country. Pravastatin did not reduce either all-cause mortality or coronary heart disease events compared to "usual care."

The statins were produced because spectacular Nobel Prize-winning science (by Konrad Bloch, Michael Brown, Joe Goldstein, and others) pointed the way. Their development is a triumph of applied biochemistry. However, the "translational" science, which seeks clinical effectiveness, is nearly as disappointing as the basic science is illuminating. Statins have a crucial role to play in the treatment of a few rare genetic disorders of cholesterol metabolism, and a defensible role in secondary prevention – averting a second heart attack. In primary prevention, however, with its potentially huge market of well people, statins should be viewed as a false start and an object lesson. Here, billions of dollars of profit are at stake for most of the major pharmaceutical firms. Marketing dollars flow into the coffers of advertising firms, professional organizations, "thought leaders" among cardiologists and endocrinologists, prescribing physicians, political war chests, and political action committees (PACs). Several voices have decried this marketing campaign, and several organizations have tried to dampen the enthusiasm. For example, the American College of Physicians weighed in on the debate on cholesterol screening and treatment in 1996 with conservative guidelines. Today, in the United States, however, cholesterol screening is considered good medicine, with cardiologists often bemoaning the fact that it is difficult to get patients to take their prescribed statins consistently over long periods.

The fact that cardiologists like statins more than their patients do shows how non-compliance can be "homeostatic" – a term coined by Harvard professor Walter Bradford Cannon in his 1932 treatise, *Wisdom of the Body*, to capture the insights that biological systems contain mechanisms to maintain stability when faced with disturbance. The idea is of a kind of force/counterforce, leading to stability. By suggesting that "non-compliance can be homeostatic," I am acknowledging those circumstances where the advice is unfounded or the prescription is unhelpful.

SYNDROME X

The hypothesis that cholesterol and various lipids are atherogenic, predisposing a person to atherosclerosis and therefore to heart attacks and stroke, has been around for over fifty years. Lipid metabolism has challenged generations of investigators.

This challenge won't go away, nor should it, for lipid metabolism harbours secrets relevant to coronary artery disease and to atherosclerosis elsewhere. The same even holds for cholesterol metabolism. After all, if you have already had one heart attack, lowering blood cholesterol is of measurable effectiveness in preventing another. If you are in the subset of patients already ill from atherosclerotic coronary artery disease, the benefit/risk ratio of pharmacologically manipulating your cholesterol metabolism justifies the intervention. If you are not in that subset, if you are not even a patient and still well in spite of whatever atherosclerosis you harbour, the effects of manipulating your cholesterol metabolism are too puny to discern reliably and, therefore, not worth your while. There are lipids and lipoproteins, many involved in cholesterol metabolism, which are also playing a part in the pathogenesis of atherosclerosis. They are slight, though independent, markers of the likelihood that you will suffer a heart attack. However, the data we have on pharmaceutical agents that manipulate these markers to our benefit is less impressive than what we have just dissected for cholesterol.

There are several reasons why all this "translational" effort seems to be going nowhere quickly. First, as I discussed in the introduction to Part One, in an advanced, industrialized country, at least 75 per cent of the hazard to longevity can be captured with measures of socioeconomic status (SES) and job satisfaction. These are sociopolitical realities that operate whether you behave in a manner adverse to your health and whether you have biological risk factors for earlier death. Health-adverse behaviours and the known biological risk factors are vying to take their toll on the other 25 per cent of your likelihood of living to old age, and they do so in an intergrated fashion. It is challenging to separate these specific elements of proximate-cause epidemiology one from the other or to manipulate them in isolation to your benefit. Perhaps that's because the elements of proximate-cause epidemiology are not so independent.

The possibility that the biological factors could integrate was recognized some years ago. It was suggested that a particular combination was so likely to result in cardiovascular disaster that it deserved designation and became known as "Syndrome X." Today, Syndrome X is generally called the "metabolic syndrome." The hallmarks are abdominal obesity, decreased insulin sensitivity leading to adult onset diabetes, abnormalities in blood lipids associated with high blood cholesterol, and hypertension. The full-blown extremes of the metabolic syndrome are alarming in terms of the 25 per cent risk to your longevity that can be ascribed to biological proximate causes; because it is atherogenic and diabetogenic, it predisposes individuals to heart attacks, renal failure, strokes, and other fatal events. The metabolic syndrome is often augmented by tobacco abuse, and it is far more likely to afflict people who are already marked by their lower socioeconomic status in advanced societies.

In 2001 an expert panel, convened by the National Institutes of Health (NIH), took a stab at criteria for the metabolic syndrome. To qualify, they said, individuals had to have three or more of the following:

- a waist circumference greater than 102 cm (40 inches) in men and 88 cm (35 inches) in women;
- hypertriglyceridemia defined as 150 mg/dl or more;
- low high-density lipoprotein (HDL) cholesterol defined as less than 40 mg/dl in men and 50 mg/dl in women;
- high blood pressure defined as 130/85 or more; and
- high fasting glucose defined as 110 mg/dl or more.

If you use these criteria, the age-adjusted prevalence of the metabolic syndrome in the United States is 23.7 per cent. For those aged sixty to sixty-nine, the prevalence is 43.5 per cent. Furthermore, the prevalence is comparable in white men, white women, and African American women, but lower in African American men. That's very peculiar epidemiology. Nearly all other studies probing associations of race/ethnicity with risk to longevity favour the white population over the African American (although these putative associations with race/ethnicity are really associations with socioeconomic status and probably have little to do with race/ethnicity itself* – with the possible exception of birth weight). Not only are the associations with ethnicity peculiar but the prevalence is striking. Do you really think that 43 per cent of Americans in their sixties should be medicalized as having the metabolic syndrome? Could it be that this definition is nonsense? After all, it is certain that more Americans are living longer despite their putative metabolic syndrome. Maybe robustness in body configuration, or habitus, and in metabolism is responsible for improving longevity, and not a curse. In fact, the less robust among the elderly live less long. A recent analysis of the risks to hearts and lives from the metabolic syndrome in Finnish men suggests that the term should be reserved for individuals in the top quarter of the population as defined by the NIH expert panel, since little risk was established for the remainder.

Full blown, the metabolic syndrome is easy to spot and its victims are not well people – not for long. It is spotting the incomplete syndrome and the early stages in the well population that is our next contentious topic. If you exhibit a little bit of the elements of the metabolic syndrome, should you be marked, marketed, and segregated as a ticking time bomb? Do the data on Finnish men generalize to other populations and to women? Let's examine the epidemiology of three attributes in the criteria: obesity, diabetes, and hypertension.

---

*After a century of presumption and assumption, modern science is finally deconstructing the construct of "race." There are genetic differences between populations with differing ancestral continents of origin. However, the genomic similarities are far more striking than the differences. Furthermore, in an outbred population such as the citizenry of the United States, the genomic differences are further blurred. Ethnic and racial labelling is on the shakiest of genetic grounds. The labels should be used with caution so as not to reinforce untenable stereotypes or to mask the sociocultural variables that are far more influential in terms of longevity and other health outcomes.

Body Mass Index

The Body Mass Index (BMI or Quatelet index) describes the heft of a person, taking into account both weight and height. The calculation is simple: weight in kilograms divided by the square of height in metres. So if you weigh 100 kg (about 220 pounds) and you're 2 metres tall (about 6 feet), your BMI = 100/4 = 25. BMI is a risk factor for dying before your time. But, like all the risk factors that are elements of the metabolic syndrome, the relationship between BMI and longevity is not linear; it is U-shaped. Some of the curves describing the relationship between proximate-cause and mortal hazard are more J-shaped than U-shaped, but none are linear. Here's a prototype curve for people in the community, plotting increasing likelihood of death before their time against increasing BMI.

U

BMI →

This graphic means that at a very high BMI and at a very low BMI, your likelihood of dying too soon increases dramatically. If your BMI exceeds 30, you have the disease "morbid obesity" and you are no longer a well person. If your BMI is very low, you have either anorexia nervosa or some yet to be diagnosed inflammatory, neoplastic, metabolic, or infectious disease. Regardless, you're in trouble. Between very high and very low, increasing BMI is a very gentle risk factor. It is somewhat less gentle if you carry discordant weight in your belly. Divide the circumference of your waist by the circumference at your hips. The greater your gut-butt ratio is over 1.0 for a man and 0.9 for a woman, the greater your risk for dying before your time. But you are still on the gentle upward slope of the base of the U-shaped curve until you are approaching a BMI of 30. If SES is taken into account, the slope is gentle indeed.

Perhaps the small risk, and therefore the limited potential yield, rather than the usual explanation of recidivism, explains the disappointing results of all those trials of weight loss. Most trials of weight loss are plagued by non-compliance. In fact, there is a hint that recurrent recidivism – "yo-yo" weight loss or weight cycling – is more likely to cost you time on earth than if you left the excess weight alone. And what of the hype that obesity is a new American epidemic? True, the average weight of Americans is increasing – but the average life expectancy is also increasing. That combination should engender cognitive dissonance for all those in public health policy who want the masses to vie for a place in the valley of the U-shaped curve. "Normal body weight" is a social construction. As long as we stay away from the sides of the U-shaped curve, we are not faced with escalating mortal hazard. To argue otherwise is to pervert science. Defining obesity short of the steep slope creates a vast marketplace for unnecessary and unproven remedies.

Blood Sugar

Blood sugar also has a U-shaped curve, though asymmetric. Few well people suffer very low blood sugar, hypoglycemia. Nearly all who feel weak or feel faint at times do not have "low blood sugar," so there is no benefit in medicalizing them for it. If we exclude people on insulin therapy, or people who have had gastric surgery, hypoglycemia is very rare. It is one sign of a pancreatic tumour that secretes insulin or, if it occurs a few hours after a meal, it may presage full-blown diabetes. Our endocrine system generally ensures that we don't suffer hypoglycemia, even if we nearly starve to death. So the U-shaped curve rises sharply at the low end, but the risk for premature death rises very gradually towards the high end of the distribution. Furthermore, aging broadens the curve, so that the valley sets at a higher blood sugar. "Normal" blood sugar is age dependent.

Who has diabetes? If you don't make insulin, you are not a well person. You have Type 1 diabetes and, without insulin therapy, you will soon die. Type 1 diabetes usually starts in childhood or young adulthood. Your blood sugar (glucose) will escalate, but the glucose will not be able to enter the cells of most of your organs without insulin. Those cells will go to extremes in attempting to use alternative energy sources, and you will be worse off as a result. If you are to survive with Type 1 diabetes, you must inject yourself with insulin from the onset of your illness. The more meticulously you administer insulin therapy, attempting to keep your blood sugar normal all the time, the more risk you run of hypoglycemia, which puts you at cognitive and mortal risk. But the tradeoff makes sense if the vascular complications of Type 1 diabetes are postponed.

The landmark study suggesting this vascular benefit used "surrogate" measures of outcome – measures that may not be directly important to you, but are sensitive to change, readily detectable, and likely to presage events that are important. The study found that meticulous control of the blood sugar of patients with Type 1 diabetes will delay the development of changes in the eyes, delay the tendency of the kidneys to leak trace amounts more of protein into the urine than normal, and protect the peripheral nerves from damage (neuropathy). These changes all reflect damage to small vessels – microcirculatory disease – and the data suggests that this microcirculatory damage results from the tissues being bathed in fluids high in glucose. The data that meticulous control of blood glucose postpones damage to large vessels is suggestive, but not as compelling. Yet it is the larger-vessel (macrovascular) atherosclerotic disease associated with heart attacks, strokes, and peripheral vascular disease that often ravages patients with Type 1 diabetes decades before others in their birth cohort.

Ever since the discovery of insulin there has been a debate as to whether tight control in Type 1 diabetes was worth the trouble and the risk of hypoglycemia. With the surrogate measures in hand and the suggestive data about postponing coronary artery disease, that debate is largely stilled. But it's too early to make a general statement that meticulous insulin dosing that normalizes the blood sugar reduces the probability of blindness, amputations, coronary artery disease, and renal failure. Medical wisdom is arguing for tight control on that basis so patients will not have missed out should the day come when outcome measures that are not surrogate prove that the medical wisdom was prescient.

I am offering this précis on Type 1 diabetes because it colours all thinking about high blood sugar, or hyperglycemia, in people who do make insulin – people labelled as having Type 2 diabetes (also called adult onset diabetes mellitus, AODM, or non-insulin dependent diabetes mellitus, NIDDM). In fact, such people make more insulin than normal, but it appears to be less effective. People with Type 2 diabetes are usually identified in mid-life or later and are at increased risk for the same vascular complications as the Type 1 patients, though the risk plays out much later in life. These people can be found on the upward slope of the asymmetric U-shaped curve for blood sugar. Where is the cut-off to abnormal, to Type 2 diabetes? Shouldn't the cut-off be adjusted for age? After all, the older you are, the more likely your blood sugar is elevated, but the less likely hyperglycemia will have time to deprive you of your longevity. Do we know that if we declare a cut-off and treat the hyperglycemia so defined, we will advantage these people? Very few hyperglycemic well people know they are hyperglycemic. Some urinate more frequently, but that's a fact of life for many aging men and women, hyperglycemic or not. The real issue is whether we can protect the hyperglycemic well people from the atherogenic vascular disease that leads to death before their time.

Several august panels, speaking for equally august professional bodies, are convinced that we can and, therefore, we should be more liberal with the cut-off. Consequently, the cut-off is progressively lowered by consensus. It follows that the prevalence of Type 2 diabetes is escalating. If we keep lowering the cut-off, soon all of us will age into Type 2 diabetes, and even more will be labelled as having the metabolic syndrome. The public health world is alarming us about yet another epidemic that it is helping to create simply by changing the labelling rules. Screening programs are advised. And, in parallel with the reasoning for treating Type 1 diabetes, meticulous management of blood sugar is called for, in this case resorting to pills designed to increase the efficiency of the patients' own insulin responsiveness before resorting to insulin therapy. These pills, called oral hypoglyce-mic agents, were first introduced some fifty years ago. This area is another hot spot of pharmaceutical development; second-generation and third-generation oral hypoglycemic agents are marketed along with new agents, and much more is in develop-ment. This enormous marketplace ranks with statins and, as we shall see, the anti-hypertensive agents. Here, too, the advisers to the medical associations and the members of the panels often have financial ties to the marketplace, one way or another. Nonetheless, they are convinced they are doing right to phar-macologically stem the tide of Type 2 diabetes, and they have convinced most payers, most providers, the lay press, and most patients who are told that their blood sugar is high.

My reflexive cynicism was planted some thirty-five years ago by the first major randomized controlled trial of an oral hypo-glycemic, obviously a first-generation agent. That agent was com-pared to diet therapy and insulin therapy in a multi-centre trial. The subjects taking the first-generation oral hypoglycemic agent were likely to die *sooner* than the other two groups. This famous trial has been used ever since to illustrate errors in design and data analysis. It had serious flaws and may or may not have led to an incorrect conclusion. Besides, very few trials of oral hypo-glycemic agents since have been powered to consider such dramatic, definitive outcomes as death. Most are looking at surrogate outcomes to generate the data on which the FDA bases the decision to license the product for sale as a prescription pharmaceutical. Nagging doubts continued in the diabetes research and treatment community until 1998, when those doubts were largely laid to rest by publication in *Lancet* of the UK Prospective Diabetes Study (UKPDS).

The stated intent of the study was to determine whether improved blood glucose control did more than manage surro-gate measures. Did it advantage, or disadvantage, the patient with Type 2 diabetes in terms of macrovascular disease and its ravages, including heart attacks and death? This study bears scrutiny. The fact that the investigators, the UKPDS Group, had the temerity to undertake such a study is remarkable in and of itself. They couldn't recruit subjects with long-standing hyper-glycemia who were at greatest risk of vascular catastrophe and expect a fair test of the hypothesis that treatment was beneficial; if there were no benefit, it would be argued that the testing had begun too late. To stand even a remote chance of an interpretable result requires enrolling and following a large, relatively young population for a long time. Otherwise there is too little likelihood of untoward outcomes in the control group to expect to be able to discern an effect in the experimental groups. This multi-centre, practice-based study started enrolling the almost 4,000 newly diagnosed patients with Type 2 diabetes in the 1970s. To qualify for enrolment, patients had to be forty-eight to sixty years old with fasting blood glucose levels of 110–270 after three months of dieting. The patients were nearly all white, a third male, with an average BMI of 28. About a third smoked, and 20 per cent were sedentary. On average they had normal blood pressure, though a third were considered hypertensive and were enrolled in an embedded second study of controlling both blood sugar and blood pressure. We know nothing of their socioeconomic status (SES), a critical confounder. They were randomized so that a third received "conventional" therapy, and the remainder, "intensive" therapy. The "conventional" group attended clinics every three months to receive advice and encouragement from a dietician. The intensive group was further randomized to receive insulin therapy, a first-generation hypoglycemic agent, or a second-generation hypoglycemic agent. Patients were followed an average of ten years. The study closed in September 1997.

The UKPDS Group are not naïve investigators. To the contrary, they were prepared to apply all that biostatistics could offer to challenges such as cross-over, drop-out, missing data, non-compliance, and treatment failure. Some of the findings are strikingly disconcerting. It is clear that the intensive therapies caused weight gain, and that the intensive hypoglycemic therapies reduced blood glucose, sometimes to the extent that there was an impressive increase in episodes of symptomatic hypoglycemia. Some of the findings are disconcertingly marginal.

There is a suggestion that intensive therapies decreased the like-lihood of some microvascular complications, notably the surrogate measures of leakage of protein from blood vessels in the retina or in the kidney. However, this effect did not translate into fewer patients suffering from kidney or eye damage. Intensive therapy did not alter the likelihood of peripheral neuropathy. It is also abundantly clear that there was no advantage from intensive therapies in terms of macrovascular complications – no decrease in heart attacks, strokes, or important peripheral vascular disease, including amputations. And there was no decrease in all-cause or in diabetes-specific mortality.

Ten years of intensive therapy offered no real advantage for 1,000 middle-aged hyperglycemic people. So why would anyone declare the UKPDS supportive of intensive therapy, including intensive therapy with oral hypoglycemics? Is it because the sur-rogate measures moved in the right direction? Wasn't the ratio-nale of undertaking the UKPDS in the first place to demonstrate benefit beyond surrogate measures? How about the weight gain, a surrogate measure that does not bode well? From my perspective, the UKPDS is an argument for "conventional" ther-apy, not pharmaceutical interventions. Furthermore, there is good reason to be wary of the next generation of hypoglycemic agents, even if they are more effective in terms of surrogate outcomes. One such agent, triglitazone, which offers a new way to enhance endogenous insulin efficiency, has already been withdrawn from the market because of liver toxicity. Physicians should pause before they leap to prescribe similar drugs as soon as they are released.

The UKPDS Group published a secondary analysis in 2000, using the same data to derive an association that is more con-sistent with their preconceived notion that treating the high blood glucose in Type 2 diabetes treats the patient in some mean-ingful way. The secondary analysis was based on the fact that some of the patients responded more readily and completely than others to whatever their treatment and, therefore, were less hyperglycemic over time. The secondary analysis demonstrates that the greater the exposure to hyperglycemia over time, the higher the incidence of microvascular and macrovascular events, including all-cause and diabetes-related death. However, this secondary analysis is "observational" – it defines a relationship. This relationship itself might reflect some other unmeasured risk factor (SES, for example). Furthermore, the authors' assertion that reducing exposure to hyperglycemia might reduce risk is admittedly hypothetical. It seems a tenuous hypothesis on which to base the present massive investment in treatment.

Hypertension

Hypertension, the third component of the metabolic syndrome, also has a J-shaped curve. No doubt the treatment of severe hypertension is to the advantage of patients, although life expectancy does not fully normalize; it just trends in that direction. There have been dozens of enormous, costly randomized controlled trials of treating mild hypertension with various pharmaceuticals, seeking evidence for effectiveness beyond merely the lowering of the blood pressure. It is a daunting literature and quite telling. The likelihood of important benefits from anti-hypertensive therapy for mild hypertension across these trials is highly varied but never dramatic. In fact, the vast majority demonstrates no change in mortality as a result of treatment. There is a decrease in the likelihood of strokes in a few, and of heart attacks in still fewer. Two of these trials are object lessons:

• MR FIT is an acronym for the Multiple Risk Factor Intervention Trial, a famous multi-centre US trial initiated in 1973 with the screening of 361,662 men aged thirty-three to forty-seven years. Most were followed as late as 1990. Much was measured, and many papers were published. Embedded in this experience early on were trials of anti-hypertensive agents – obviously older agents used in a "step" fashion that begins with the milder drugs. The surprise finding was that hypertensive patients who were treated with gentle diuretics fared poorly, an observation that led to several creative explanations. It is likely that the excess mortality reflected dose-dependent drug toxicity (electrolyte disturbances), although I would not discount randomization errors. Regardless, it is worth emphasizing that treating well people with mild hypertension with drugs has a disconcertingly tight benefit/risk ratio. No well person should be persuaded otherwise. A recent analysis of the MR FIT cohort, sixteen years after inception, documents that socioeconomic status overwhelms and subsumes all the measured biological risk factors for all-cause mortality as well as most other mortal and illness (morbid) end-points.

- It has become clear that gentle anti-hypertensive therapy will benefit the elderly with systolic hypertension – and that's the majority of the elderly. In fact, this is the only group of well patients with mild hypertension I feel confident I am helping by treating their mild hypertension. The elderly are likely to enjoy a meaningful benefit in cardiovascular morbidity, a meaningful decrease in the incidence of stroke, and perhaps a little extra longevity. However, I can justify only a gentle and inexpensive single-drug regimen. Furthermore, another randomized controlled trial, the TONE study, demonstrated that some weight reduction in the more robust, and some reduction of salt intake in the less robust, is as effective among the elderly as gentle diuretic therapy. That finding gives the elderly a choice. The same pertains to the less elderly. In the PREMIER trial, 800 mildly hypertensive adults with a mean age of fifty were randomized to various behaviour modifications. Behaviour modification in the PREMIER trial is as effective in lowering blood pressure as low-dose combination pharmaceuticals, if the recent meta-analysis of 354 randomized double-blind placebo controlled trials pertains to these drug combinations.

Still, the medical literature advocates the use of drugs in the treatment of well younger people with mild hypertension – a medical literature scarred by vested interest. The brouhaha over the effectiveness of a class of anti-hypertensive drugs, the calcium channel antagonists, is instructive. The controversy commenced with the publication of a trial in the *Journal of the American Medical Association* purporting to demonstrate increased likelihood of

myocardial infarction, or heart attacks, in patients treated with
a particular calcium channel blocker. In the next year, the medical literature was peppered with nearly seventy commentaries,
some with multiple authors, taking a stand on this issue. It turns
out that the authors who supported the use of calcium channel
blockers as anti-hypertensive agents were far more likely to admit
a financial arrangement with pharmaceutical companies that
sold these agents. Likewise, authors who took a stand against
using the calcium channel blockers were far more likely to have
a vested interest in pharmaceutical firms that sold competing
classes of anti-hypertensive drugs. Although the association with
increased mortality that initiated the brouhaha proved irrepro-
ducible in subsequent trials, it is sensible to be wary of all claims
of pharmaceutical benefit for well people who have mild hypertension – particularly of benefit from newer, more expensive
agents. The same ALLHAT trial I mentioned above, which
showed no benefit from treatment with pravastatin, also sought
a differential benefit across classes of anti-hypertensive agents.
Over 33,000 participants age fifty-five or older with mild hypertension were randomized to treatment with a standard and inexpensive diuretic, a drug of the calcium channel blocker class,
or a drug of the angiotensin-converting enzyme (ACE) inhibitor class. Those treated with the old-fashioned inexpensive
diuretic were less likely to suffer a major cardiovascular event
during five years of follow-up. Maybe, as MR FIT suggests, they
would have been even better off not treated.

We've now examined the elements of the metabolic syndrome
and dissected the degree to which they are noxious. In each
instance, a well person needs to be up the limb of the U-shaped
curve before the hazard is clinically meaningful enough to warrant being labelled obese, diabetic, or hypertensive. In each
instance, the data that suggests we can intervene effectively,
short of the extremes, is tenuous at best. What about people at
the extremes? The data is suggestive – and is bolstered by a series
of articles that examines the benefits of treating the hypertension of a patient with both Type 2 diabetes and hypertension.

It is clear that hypertension and diabetes are synergistic evils. Much of this information derives from secondary analyses of many of the hypertension drug trials I have already referred to. Investigators went back to the data to extract the subjects who had coincident Type 2 diabetes and hypertension and found that most of the effectiveness demonstrated in these trials is restricted to the stratum of hypertensive patients who were also diabetic. That includes the influential SHEP trial; there, the annual cardiovascular event rate among 4,149 non-diabetic elderly patients decreased from about 3.5 per cent to 2.5 per cent after treating their systolic hypertension, but for the 583 with Type 2 diabetes it decreased from just over 6 per cent to about 4 per cent, a slightly more credible benefit.

The analysis of the UKPDS trial is even more illuminating, particularly since, embedded in that trial, were some 4,000 patients with hypertension and Type 2 diabetes. After a complex allocation scheme, 1,000 were randomized to either tight or less tight blood pressure control. The incidence of almost all end-points was lower in the patients whose blood pressure was tightly controlled. For example, if the systolic blood pressure was maintained below 120 mm of mercury, there were 7 deaths per 1,000 people per year. If the systolic blood pressure could not be maintained below 160, there were 30 deaths per 1,000 persons per year. About 13 people in 1,000 (1.3%) with diabetes and hypertension who would have died that year, therefore, would live to die another year. Suppose I grant, begrudgingly, that we can measure this difference. It is the order of magnitude of benefit, consistently, in four other trials similar to UKPDS. They, too, have acronyms: ABCD, MDRD, HOT, and AASK. However, to achieve the blood pressure reduction goal in all these trials, the patient was not on a simple, gentle regimen. To the contrary, these patients were taking, on average, three anti-hypertensive agents, and each agent had its own set of problems.

For patients with Type 2 diabetes and hypertension, given the tradeoffs and uncertainties, the decision to treat or not to treat with hypoglycemic agents is easier. The decision to treat with multiple anti-hypertensive drugs is challenging and requires a dialogue. Most patients who have had the opportunity to build a relationship of trust with their physician will ask: "What would you do, Doc?" Thanks to the ALLHAT data, prescribing an inexpensive, gentle diuretic is an appealing option. I might even be tempted to advise changing lifestyle, although to do so is a cop-out, since the science supporting that advice is as tenuous as the science that documents compliance with the advice.

THE EUPHEMISM OF LIFESTYLE CHANGES

Literature such as we've reviewed provides fodder for my cynicism. The "science" of epidemiology often seems to promulgate the scare of the week and the cure of the month. Epidemiology has lost its way. In fact, epidemiology may lose its credibility, given its tendency to declare last month's "good" this month's "evil." The modern mission of epidemiology is to probe for associations between exposures and health effects. It has enlightened us about the association between smoking and lung cancer, inhalation of certain types of asbestos fibres and mesathelioma, alcohol consumption and motor vehicle accidents. Buoyed by such success, it is now probing for associations between exposures that are difficult to define and health effects that clearly have multiple causal associations. Epidemiology is acquiring near religious belief that statistical modelling is a match for any degree of variability and uncertainty in the definition of exposure, and that imperious p-values are a match for discerning, as specific, even a tiny health effect.

We've examined the Pravachol trial as an example of the pitfalls in the first instance, and the UKPDS trial as an example of the pitfalls in the second. These were randomized controlled trials in which the investigators had some control over the exposure, and still the results are equivocal and the authors' interpretations, unconvincing. Nonetheless, these randomized controlled trials stand far above observational studies. Epidemiology fails when it tries to tease minor exposures and minor health effects by observing all the variability that is humanity. Biases in these studies and confounders await any epidemiologist who is trying to tease minor events and influences out of the complexity of life. Condemnation awaits any epidemiologist who is willing to analyze data with the goal of supporting a preconceived notion (data dredging) rather than testing a hypothesis. Most disconcerting is the fact that much of this epidemiology is generated in trials that are supported by companies that are purveying, or wish to purvey, the pharmaceutical under study. Recent analyses of the published results of such industry-sponsored trials document systematic biases that favour the drug when compared to trials of the same drug sponsored by other sources. The Last Well Person can take little for granted.

It's time to admit limitations and call a halt to pseudo-science. Data dredging, bias, and confounding are tarnishing the credibility of modern epidemiology. Data dredging is the exercise of reworking data analyses till the result fits a preconceived notion. Bias is a systematic error that creeps into the way in which the study is conducted – allocating sicker patients to a control group, for instance, will make the drug being tested seem more effective. Confounding is the influence of unmeasured or immeasurable variables. All three create problems. Data dredging is condemnable – the analysis to be performed must be decided and honed before the study commences. Bias is excusable only if every effort has been made to avoid it. And confounders are, by definition, always lurking. For that reason, only robust results should have influence, and statistically significant absolute differences of less than 2 per cent or even 3 per cent should be published only so they can be ignored. Trumpeting such results in the scientific literature, let alone the lay press, is unacceptable.

Let's take the example of the hype over the salutary nature of a diet rich in fish, plying us with omega-3 fatty acids. As is true for many of the putatively life-saving diets that bombard our world, someone noted that peoples elsewhere are living longer and have diets that seem distinctive. The dearth of atherosclerotic disease afflicting the Eskimos of Greenland and the longevity of rural native Japanese, combined with the fact that their diets are rich in seafood, was held up as more than coincidence. No one seems concerned that these are genetically distinctive populations living in countries with distinctive socio-economic structures. The notions seem credible that eating fish, or a Mediterranean diet, or green vegetables, or less meat, or more carbohydrate, or less saturated fats, or whatever promises the fountain of youth. To test the inference with a randomized controlled trial in a well population is prohibitive. It's daunting enough to test a pharmaceutical, where you can administer pills that contain either the active agents or a placebo, never mind controlling the diets of half the sample for decades, waiting to see how many die. Even modern epidemiology has no such hubris. But modern epidemiology comes close with its belief that it can test inferences about subtle risk just by observing large populations at work and play.

Take the example of the famous Nurses' Health Study based at Harvard. In 1976, 121,700 registered nurses, all women between the ages of thirty and fifty-five and nearly all white, were enrolled in the study, with an extensive questionnaire probing details about their lifestyle and medical history. Every two years since, follow-up questionnaires have been sent to update information and identify new major illnesses. In 1980, 1984, 1986, 1990, and 1994 the women were asked how often they had consumed particular foods, on average, during the previous year, with a scale ranging from "almost never" to "six or more times per day." During sixteen years of follow-up, amounting to 1,307,157 years of life that 100,000 responding nurses lived, almost 500 deaths were ascribed to coronary heart disease and 1,000 suffered non-fatal heart attacks – i.e., only 0.5 per cent of the cohort was dead, and another 1 per cent had suffered a non-fatal heart attack over the course of sixteen years. Even if every one of these 1,500 women avoided fish all their lives, and the remaining 98,500 women ate fish often, I would still be sceptical. I would wonder what else was going on that we weren't measuring. Of course, the exposure was not so binary, it was not uniform year by year, and it cannot be measured reliably (short of a food diary, the recall of dietary habits for a year is problematic). In fact, forty-one of the women who suffered a fatal heart attack recalled eating fish less than once per month, and twenty-five more than once a month, and the remaining 400 fatalities were spread out between these extremes of fish consumption.

By inspection, the raw data looks unpromising if you believe that eating fish is good for you. The investigators were undaunted, however, and statistically modelled the data to account for differences in age, BMI, cigarette smoking, hypertension, blood cholesterol, Type 2 diabetes, and the like to come up with relative risks that suggested a statistically significant protective effect of eating fish. The absolute reduction in risk was minuscule and it was not apparent till the data was massaged statistically. Such modelling of small effects is susceptible to confounding. For example, "job satisfaction" has been an issue for the nursing profession, and lack thereof is a mortal risk that was not considered in the statistical modelling. But the investigators are enamoured of their methodology. They even estimated the content of omega-3 fatty acids that was being consumed and advised we all partake. Similarly, the pitfall of the unmeasured confounder may explain the tiny survival benefit observed for those among 22,000 Greek adults who adhered more tightly to a "Mediterranean diet" over the course of forty-four months of observation. Multiple confounders were taken into account, but not socioeconomic status.

Other cohort studies similar to the Nurses' Health Study have examined the relation of leisure-time physical activity to all-cause mortality and cardiac outcomes. These studies find an inverse relationship between activity and mortality. All these studies factor in biological risk factors and health adverse behaviours such as tobacco abuse. But they do not consider socioeconomic status. Who is likely to spend an hour or two each week exercising for fun? Who is likely to choose to walk the stairs rather than take an elevator? Is it the advantaged person whose work is not physically demanding? How many blue-collar production workers or materials handlers or field hands want to ride an exercise bicycle after work?

I don't want to leave you with the impression that all observational studies are doomed to be irrelevant or that the Nurses'

Health Study has no redeeming features. On the contrary, it has been the source of several important insights. For example, it was shown that nurses who chose to have silicon breast implants were no more likely than their peers to suffer rheumatoid arthritis or any other major systemic rheumatic disease. The observational design is a match for that insight because both the exposure (breast implants) and the health effect (systemic rheumatic diseases) are well defined. The design is even a match for probing for biological risk factors for death or myocardial infarction, although there are challenges to defining the exposure (e.g., blood sugar, cholesterol, or blood pressure) when the measure can vary considerably over the course of observation. However, trying to define dietary exposures, stressful exposures, level of physical activity, or other aspects of the fabric of daily life over sixteen years of observation requires multiple suppositions and approximations. Any investigator or funding agency with the temerity to try is begging to be wrong.

However, there are studies that are designed to ask some lifestyle questions in a way that might provide meaningful insights. Most examine population at high risk for the particular health effect and are experimental in design. They are usually randomized controlled trials and demanding of resources. But they are less susceptible to confounding and bias. More than not, these studies trump the notions based on observational data. That's why a voluminous observational literature suggests that antioxidant vitamins protect you from cardiac disease, but the experimental literature finds no such benefit.

Let me mention three randomized controlled trials that tested the effectiveness of lifestyle alterations that the investigators thought should benefit the subjects. All relied on surrogate measures of outcome. All inform our common sense and influence the thinking of the members of committees convened to advise on the common good.

- In 1997 the DASH collaborative research group published a trial on the effects of dietary patterns on blood pressure. Nearly 500 normal adults were enrolled. For three weeks they were fed an average American diet, low in fruits and vegetables. For the next eight weeks they were randomized to continue the control diet, eat a diet rich in fruits and vegetables, or a diet rich in fruits and vegetables but reduced in saturated and total fats. Sodium intake and body weight were maintained at constant levels. The experimental diets were associated with a lowering of blood pressure, particularly in subjects whose blood pressures were in the upper range.

- In 2001 the Finnish Diabetes Prevention Study Group published a multi-centre randomized controlled study of the effectiveness of lifestyle alteration in preventing type 2 diabetes. They enrolled some 500 middle-aged people who were clearly overweight (average BMI = 31) and had impaired glucose tolerance as well. The intervention group each had seven sessions with dieticians the first year, and quarterly thereafter, to instruct, urge, and monitor compliance with an exercise regimen and a diet tailored to be high in fibre, lower in calories, and low in saturated fats. The control group received educational material and instruction at entry and, annually, for the three years of the study. The intervention group lost more weight than the control group, and had less progression in the degree of glucose intolerance.

- The Diabetes Prevention Program Research Group published the results of its three-year trial in 2002. It had recruited over 3,000 overweight people (average BMI = 34) with mild glucose intolerance. These people were randomly assigned to receive routine care plus a placebo, routine care plus metformin, or an intensive program aimed at modifications in lifestyle. Metformin is an interesting hypoglycemic agent that is unique in not having weight gain as a common side effect. The study originally included a fourth limb on triglitazone, but the FDA withdrew that drug in 1998 because of liver toxicity. The intensive program started with a sixteen-session curriculum taught on a one-to-one basis and covering diet, exercise, and behaviour modification. Monthly individual and group sessions for reinforcement followed. After three years, more impressive progression in glucose intolerance was demonstrated in the placebo group compared to the other two, with the lowest incidence in the lifestyle group. Both intervention groups lost weight in the first year, but the metformin group was nearly back to baseline by the end of the study, and the lifestyle group well on its way towards baseline.

Despite the wealth of research data at our disposal, we continue to speculate about the best lifestyle. Vegetables, fibre, carbohydrates, fats (saturated or not), exercise (aerobic or not), and the like seem to pass in and out of "public health" favour more rapidly than the phases of the moon. In September 2002 an expert panel, convened by the National Institute of Medicine in Washington, proclaimed "New Dietary Guidelines," expanding the recommended daily intake of carbohydrates and fat, and doubling the amount of exercise recommended daily from thirty minutes to one hour. I am forced to wonder if all this is missing the forest for the trees. No doubt lifestyle can influence such surrogate outcomes as glucose metabolism and BMI. However, there remains much doubt as to whether the dietary particulars or exercise components are as important as the sense of community that is required if any such lifestyle intervention is to be successful. We will revisit this notion in detail in Part Two.

3

You and Your Colon

About 1 per cent of the North American population dies each year – approximately 3 million people. The proximate cause of death for 1 million is designated as cardiovascular disease, and another 0.6 million die from cancer, or malignant neoplasms – new growths capable of invading and destroying other tissues. The great majority of cancer deaths occur well after the age of sixty-five.

Of the 600,000 cancer deaths, a quarter stem from lung cancer. About 10 per cent are from cancer that started in the colon or rectum and spread, or metastasized. Colorectal cancer is followed closely in incidence by deaths from prostate and breast cancer. This chapter considers to what lengths the well person should go to avoid death by colorectal cancer. There are options that will decrease the likelihood of acquiring colorectal cancer in the first place, and others that will decrease the likelihood of dying from colorectal cancer. However, the existence of these options does not necessarily mean they must be chosen. Rather, we need to choose those options that may result in a pleasant time on this earth, or what is commonly termed a "good quality of life." If choosing certain options does nothing more than alter the cause of dying at approximately the same time, the choices may be far less compelling. It is likely that a significant number of the older people whose death is ascribed to cardiovascular disease harboured undetected breast, prostate, or colon cancer. It is also likely that many of the older people who died from breast or prostate or colon cancer had non-malignant co-morbidities – other diseases, including cardiovascular illness – any one of which could be their ultimate cause of death. The well person wants reassurance that avoiding colon cancer is more than a futile exercise in trying to extend longevity and improve quality of life.

Colorectal cancer can be a relatively indolent disease compared with other cancers. From the time of diagnosis, the five-year survival rate is around 50 per cent, compared with 3 per cent for pancreatic cancer, 10 per cent for lung cancer, and 70 per cent for breast cancer. It follows that if you make it to the age of eighty-five without colon cancer, it's hard to imagine that any screening would be justified. At that age, you may succumb to many quite different diseases before you reach ninety. The other extreme of the age spectrum is more problematic. The death of a young person is a tragedy, regardless of the cause. If a disease-specific tragedy such as death from colon cancer could be avoided, nothing would stay our hand. However, the disease is so rare in young people that, to save a life, we would be compelled to screen the haystack looking for a very small needle. All those well young people would then be exposed to procedures and risks for little yield, and even small risks to a well population overwhelm the gain of detecting a young person with colorectal cancer. For the young well population, selective screening is offered for those whose parents or siblings may have developed colon cancer at a younger age and for those with a family history of diseases that predispose to colorectal cancer – such as genetic diseases that cause the growth of polyps.

When is the well person too young or too old to justify screening? The answer is much debated, even though it seems at first to be relatively straightforward. It could, after all, be based on an analysis of the age-dependent efficiency of the various screening options. However, there is daunting variability in the statistics that define this efficiency, variability that derives from individual differences in the biology of patients and in the proficiency of screeners. Some critical data are missing, forcing guesses and approximations. As a result, the definition of age-dependent efficiency depends on the statistics contrived for the analysis.

That is just the start of the complexity. There is also the issue of ethics. How justified is the exposure of all young well people to risks in order to spare one young person death from colorectal cancer? Most scholars and expert panels are unwilling to depart from the standard for statistical modelling in this field – a model that considers death by colorectal cancer to be the important outcome. I disagree: I want a more meaningful outcome measure, such as the number of good-quality-of-life years that would otherwise be lost to colon cancer were it not for screening. If screening spares you death by colorectal cancer but you die at about the same time from something else, was the screening valuable? Personally, I am not impressed by interventions that do no more than change the proximate cause of death. With that as my bias, I will explain how to choose whether to undergo screening for colorectal cancer.

Although financial cost is a huge issue, I don't want to be influenced by it in my argument. In this era of "managed care" – or, to be cynical, the managed transfer of wealth – many analyses are designed to assess financial cost/benefit ratios rather than other risk/benefit ratios. Recent analyses estimate $1,000 as the "cost" of colonoscopy. One British colleague put it nicely when he mused: "There's a thousand-dollar bill in every American colon. You just have to get up there and find it." But it need not be $1,000. The procedure is tedious and demands some dexterity, but it does not require more than procedure-specific training. In two controlled studies, nurse practitioners have been trained to perform colonoscopy with a proficiency indistinguishable from that of the gastroenterologists who trained them and at a fraction of the cost. In this chapter, however, I'll focus on risk/benefit considerations.

Let's start with the absurd. If we all had our colons removed at the age of fifty, we wouldn't have colon cancer. Imagine that surgeons honed their laparoscopic techniques so that they could work through tiny incisions to remove the colons of outpatients, fashion a pouch from the terminal small bowel, and attach the pouch to the rectal sphincters. Most would retain normal bowel function, the expense would be reasonable (perhaps equivalent to five or ten screening colonoscopies), and serious complications rare. Would you do it? Would you do it if gastroenterologists, laparoscopic surgeons, and august professional bodies recommended it and it was covered by your "health" insurer? Probably not: most people would consider this scenario a parody. Short of removing the hazard by removing the colon – colectomy – several screening options are available that promise to detect colon cancer before it becomes a problem. To understand the limitations of these options, however, we must first understand the enemy.

THE NATURAL HISTORY OF COLORECTAL CANCER

With some exceptions, all the tissues and organs of our bodies turn over and renew, each with an internal rhythm that allows older cells to die at the same rate as younger cells take their place. The process is elegantly orchestrated so that our tissues and organs maintain their architecture and function, lifelong, for most of us. Minor aberrancies in turnover are common and may result in benign tumours that lack any potential to spread and destroy. So long as these neoplasms do not alter the functions of the organ from which they arose, they are safe. There are other benign tumours, however, that have the potential to undergo a transformation, losing some critical features of the normal biology of their tissues of origin. Some acquire architectural characteristics that are distinctive, while the cells of others lose the need to associate with like cells in order to turn over normally. Some cells acquire the biology to be indiscriminate about their nurturing neighbourhood. If they acquire these last two features, they have the potential to take up residence elsewhere in the body, commandeering the host tissue to serve their needs. These distant explants are metastases, and their tumour of origin is a "malignant" tumour – a cancer.

Some cancers develop in a relatively predictable fashion, over longer time and through the stages already outlined. Cervical cancer, prostate cancer, and colorectal cancer may be of this type. The time that malignant neoplasms spend in a pre-invasive state is referred to as the "dwell time." There is variability in the dwell time, between tumour types and from person to person. If the dwell time of a particular tumour type is not too short, population screening can be useful. Hence, screening with cervical "Pap" smears is defensible for detecting the earliest stages of cervical cancer and intervening to remove it. Is there a similar justification for colorectal cancers, since various authors estimate the dwell time of colorectal cancer to be between one and two decades?

More aggressive and potentially lethal cancers have brief dwell times. They undergo the transformation to the biology of metastasis too quickly to permit staging or even screening. Some may arise already endowed with the potential of ready metastasis. "Breast cancer" is so heterogeneous that some tumours manifest "highly variable" biology, thereby confounding the attempts to design and interpret screening programs.

Benign tumours can be more common in the colon and rectum as we age. Most are polyps on a stalk (like a grape) and are composed of cells representative of the normal lining cells of the colon. Some grow quite large on the end of their stalk. Other benign tumours arise from the lining on a broader base and are called adenomas. Half the adenomas have distorted architecture. They also have the potential to grow in situ, even to the extent of blocking the colon and obstructing the bowel.

Colorectal cancer seems to start in some of these benign tumours. The adenomas, particularly those with distorted architecture, are most likely to transform further, so that cells that are normally restricted to the lining of the colon are observed in the deeper layers and take on the appearance of malignant cells. These cells may be on their way towards metastatic biology. However, their metastatic biology is relatively specific and they prefer to take up residence in the local lymph nodes and the liver, the sites to which blood and lymph from the colon drain. These cells generally do not use the bloodstream to metastasize widely to the lungs, brain, and elsewhere. Metastatic colorectal cancer is a chronic debilitating disease. One aspect, colonic obstruction, can be remedied surgically, though recent studies from the Mayo Clinic suggest we should stop performing radical surgery for obstruction in the frail elderly in the quest for "cure." A simple bypass procedure with a colostomy is the palliative solution.

Autopsy studies give us a reasonable idea of the age-dependent prevalence of the early stages in the evolution of colorectal cancer. About 1 per cent of people at the age of fifty have at least one polyp, and the population acquires polyps at a rate of about 1 per cent a year after this age. We also know that at the age of fifty, a person has about a 2 per cent chance of dying from colorectal cancer over the next thirty years. And we know that at the age of fifty, a person has about a 60 per cent chance of dying from all causes over the next thirty years. There's the rub.

Suppose there was a screening technique that could reduce by 60 per cent a person's chance of dying after the age of fifty from colorectal cancer. What would it mean to you? Given the nature of relative risk or relative risk reduction, that 60 per cent reduction would mean that your 2 per cent chance of dying from colorectal cancer in the next thirty years was reduced to 1.2 per cent, but your chance of dying from all cancers would not be meaningfully reduced.

That is the big picture. Some of the details are interesting enough for us to examine, but we shouldn't let these considerations cause us to lose our way. Most epidemiologists in this field, most policy makers, most gastroenterologists, and all who do colonoscopy for a living are focused on their own particular small picture. Is the 0.8 per cent reduction in risk of dying from colorectal cancer after the age of fifty a relevant statistic? Let's tackle the reliability issue first. Then we can examine our choices.

SCREENING FOR COLORECTAL CANCER BY FOBT

Fecal occult blood testing (FOBT) is a method of testing a small sample of stool for trace amounts of blood. It's indelicate, but at least it's safe. It's also inexpensive, until you start designing FOBT screening programs that involve multiple samplings from large numbers of people. FOBT has been around for generations, in spite of well-documented inherent limitations. Some polyps, particularly adenomatous polyps, and most colorectal cancers bleed, but not all of them and not all the time. This false-negative rate limits the sensitivity of FOBT and explains why most FOBT screening programs call for multiple samples. Even more factors limit the specificity, or the false-positive rate, of FOBT. First, it is normal to lose a few millilitres of blood into the bowel daily, so, if the FOBT is too sensitive, all of us will test positive. Second, there are non-cancerous lesions with a propensity to bleed – tiny fragile blood vessels and arteriovenous malformations that are common in the elderly colon. Bleeding from the mouth and throat, particularly the gums, and from gastritis and peptic ulcer disease also occurs. Finally, the FOBT is not specific for human blood; ingesting a rare steak and certain vegetables can cause a false positive.

Only in the past decade has screening for colorectal cancer by FOBT been subjected to careful scientific scrutiny. There are now four randomized controlled trials. They are all similar to the first, the Minnesota Colon Cancer Control Study, published in 1993. The cohort at inception included some 47,000 adults between the ages of fifty and eighty. They were randomized to three groups – one that had an FOBT annually, one that had an FOBT biennially, and a control group – and they were followed for thirteen years. About 90 per cent in the tested groups had at least one FOBT, and about half were fully compliant with the protocol. Over the course of the study there were some 80 deaths from colorectal cancer in the group screened annually, and about 120 in each of the biennial and control groups – a statistically significant reduction in disease-specific mortality. There was absolutely no difference, however, in all-cause mortality across the groups – about 3,300 in each group. Out of 47,000 people, to spare forty individuals over the age of fifty a death by colon cancer required identifying the true positives among the 75 per cent of those tested who had false positives. In other words, more than 20,000 people underwent a diagnostic study to determine whether the positive FOBT was a false positive or one of the forty true positives. This testing included 12,246 colonoscopies. Of these, four resulted in perforation of the colon (all requiring surgery) and eleven resulted in serious bleeding (three requiring surgery).

If we relied on FOBT as a screening method, we would have to screen about 1,000 people over the age of fifty for a decade to spare one death by colorectal cancer. In so doing, we would not affect mortality from all causes. And if we relied on colonoscopy to determine if a positive FOBT was a true or a false positive, for every person spared death by colon cancer, a person with a normal bowel would suffer a serious, non-fatal complication during diagnosis.

According to the expert panels for most of the past decade, scientific scrutiny supports having an annual FOBT. However, because of its cost and potential hazards, colonoscopy was not advised as the preferred method of determining whether positive tests were true positives indicating the presence of cancer. There was also concern about its accuracy. One study recruited 183 patients with a positive FOBT to undergo two colonoscopies by two different experienced colonoscopists on the same day. The first colonoscopist removed all the polyps and adenomas that were discovered, 289 in all. The second found another 89 that the first had missed.

Before 2000, the expert panels tended to advise flexible sigmoidoscopy to follow up on a positive FOBT. The flexible sigmoidoscope is inserted into the colon a distance of 60 centimetres; the colonoscope, in contrast, is inserted twice as far, all the way to the small intestine. The majority of colorectal cancers arise within 60 centimetres of the anus. Flexible sigmoidoscopy takes less time, requires less dexterity and fewer support personnel, and is performed without sedation (although only a gastroenterologist could imagine it is not seriously unpleasant). Most professionals agreed that an annual FOBT on three samples was advisable, relying on flexible sigmoidoscopy to verify positive tests.

In 2000, two articles appeared in the *New England Journal of Medicine*, cross-sectional studies that essentially reiterated the obvious. If you do flexible sigmoidoscopy, you will miss all cancers beyond the reach of that scope – a substantial minority. An accompanying editorial questioned why we don't just "Go the Distance." The lay medical press was already intimately involved with colorectal cancer screening because the husband of Katie Couric, the host of NBC's *Today Show*, had recently died from this disease. March 2000 was designated as "colon cancer awareness month," and a five-part documentary was aired on the *Today Show*, including Ms Couric's own colonoscopy. Before the end of 2000 Medicare decided to support colorectal cancer screening, including colonoscopy, and the American Cancer Society was pressing health insurers to the same end. The general consensus has evolved to forgo FOBT and flexible sigmoidoscopy and move directly to colonoscopy, with a frequency based on some guess at the dwell time. The zeal is such that the medical community is downplaying the possible risks associated with testing. Fortunately an article has appeared that makes the case for sparing all average-risk people under the age of fifty. In addition, the 2002 recommendations of the US Preventive Services Task Force is indecisive on the issue of colonoscopy.

As a well person over the age of fifty, how will you contend with your friend's sense of triumph at undergoing a screening colonoscopy, the common wisdom that it makes sense, the likely recommendation of your primary care physician, and the complicity of the gastroenterology community with this sophistry? As for me, I'll pass on an FOBT and forgo screening colonoscopy. I did submit in my mid-fifties to a flexible sigmoidoscopy, performed because of complications from a ruptured appendix. There were no abnormalities, so I know I am very unlikely to die before my time from colorectal cancer. I would not have cared if a polyp or two were found, so long as there was no high-risk lesion that might cost me time on earth. I don't care if I die of colorectal cancer, as long as it's my time to die anyway. You, however, will have to make up your own mind.

COLORECTAL CANCER PREVENTION

Two recent randomized placebo-controlled trials of aspirin have demonstrated a decrease in the incidence of recurrent, or

Table 3.1
Use of Aspirin for Prevention of Heart Attack and Colorectal Cancer

Outcome	Number Needed to Treat (NNT) to Prevent One Outcome	Duration of Treatment (years)
SECONDARY PREVENTION		
Recurrence of adenoma	10	2.5
Recurrence of advanced cancer	19	2.8
PRIMARY PREVENTION		
Heart attack (fatal or not)	50–250	5
Colorectal cancer	471–962	>5
Death from colorectal cancer	1,250	10–20+
ADVERSE EVENTS		
Gastrointestinal bleeding	100	1.5
Major GI haemorrhage	300–800	4–6
Haemorrhagic stroke	800	4–6

secondary, adenomas in patients who had already had an adenoma removed. Members of this group are at higher risk for colorectal cancer because they have already demonstrated that proclivity. The results show a statistically significant reduction in incidence in patients who took low doses of aspirin, compared to those taking higher doses or a placebo. The price of this attempt to avoid death from colorectal cancer, however, is the remote possibility of major gastrointestinal haemorrhaging, which has to be weighed against the small potential magnitude of benefit. Consequently, the benefit/risk ratio for prevention in someone who has never had colon cancer – primary prevention – is prohibitive, and for someone whose colon cancer has been cured – secondary prevention – it is marginal. The numbers compiled by Thomas Imperiale in table 3.1 show that. Just as trials have shown that benefit/risk ratio of aspirin therapy to try to prevent a first heart attack is not compelling, neither is it, for colorectal cancer. In both cases the use of aspirin therpary is justified for secondary prevention.

Most people, most physicians, and most endoscopists (physicians trained to slide tubes down your gullet or through your rectum in order to identify and sometimes treat pathology) have not critiqued the present situation as I have just done. We know the current approach to colorectal cancer screening is vulnerable to any alternative that makes more sense. Clinical science is not static, and screening for colorectal cancer is a topic entwined with fame and fortune. New approaches to screening are on the way, and I urge you to be very wary.

Two new approaches that are vying for acceptance are both scientifically seductive. However, both have inherent limitations that demand close inspection by you, the potential patient, even if they pass muster with the FDA.

The first tries to define, by genetic screening, more subsets of people at high enough risk to make the risk/benefit ratio of screening colonoscopy defensible. There is precedent for this approach with subsets of well people who have a family history of the genetic diseases that cause multiple polyps. For them, genetic screening is possible, and colonoscopy, if not colectomy, reasonable. The second precedent is the subset of people with a history of colon cancer in a young, first-degree relative. However, there is feverish activity trying to define genes that infer susceptibility to colorectal cancer on those of us who make up the vast majority. If you can define those at greatest risk, the risk/benefit of screening colonoscopy might favour the procedure. However, genotypes that infer slight increases in risk do not alter the risk/benefit ratio sufficiently to change our argument. To do so would require genotypes that infer considerable risk and therefore define the vast majority of people at risk. Then tens of thousands, not millions, would be subjected to screening colonoscopy annually. I doubt there is such a genetic influence. For most of us, the risk for colorectal cancer may be stochastic – the luck of the draw.

The second approach is to discover a better alternative to FOBT. For example, reagents that recognize only human blood eliminate the false positive that follows from eating a rare steak – but that discovery hardly improves FOBT. It turns out that the more malignant lesions not only bleed but shed abnormal cells and cell fragments bearing tumour-specific DNA, RNA, and protein traces. Finding these tumour-specific traces, in theory, would reduce false positives, but not false negatives (tumours that didn't shed when you sample), so specificity and sensitivity will have to be redefined. The limitation to fecal molecular screening is in the technology. All the techniques depend on chemical reagents that are unreliable. They can be rendered magnificently specific and sensitive in pure systems where there are few unknown chemicals, but much effort will be required to define how they perform when their target has to be isolated from feces sampled from millions of people. And then there's the cost of it all.

I suspect that a defensible approach to screening that spares us the risk of dying from colorectal cancer before our time will remain a will-o'-the-wisp for some time to come.

4

Breast Cancer
and How the Women's Movement
Got It Wrong

Heuristics is the branch of logic that offers the option of doing the best you can when faced with uncertainty. Medical heuristics drives all the "rules of thumb," "common practice," and "best we can offer, given the lack of evidence" statements that abound in the clinic, at the bedside, and in the lay press. It is more a reflection of preconceived notions than of refutationist science. The twentieth-century saga of breast cancer is an object lesson in medical heuristics. A compelling outcry has driven an impressive response that outpaces the evidence of benefit and, to a considerable extent, has left iatrogenicity, or harm caused by medical action, in its wake.

Breast cancer seldom countenances dispassionate or objective treatment. The topic roils with gender issues, even though it is now widely recognized that no one should be deprived of high-quality care for any reason, including gender and ethnic origins. However, the outcry to redress the gender issues by providing empathic and effective remedies carries an inherent hazard. We need to address past wrongs, but ill-thought-out attempts to do so may not benefit those who justly feel poorly served.

Radical mastectomy – the surgical removal of a cancerous breast along with the underlying muscles and the draining lymph nodes in the armpit (axilla) – provides a cautionary case study of iatrogenicity. For much of the twentieth century, medical heuristics drove the idea of a radical mastectomy to the heights of the super-radical mastectomy. Surgeons invaded the neck, chest wall, and chest cavity to extirpate every lymph node that might harbour a metastasis. This extensive surgery was not considered mutilating at the time because the scalpel was generally viewed as the instrument of cure and the conduit to longevity. Towards the end of his career in the 1960s, one of the doubters, Oliver Cope, a professor of surgery at the Massachusetts General Hospital, realized that the radical mastectomy had not discernibly improved the five-year survival of patients compared to historical controls. Earlier generations of women had the same 50 per cent survival rate over the same span of years. Yet no medical journal would publish Cope's observation after it failed "peer" review, so he settled for an article in a women's magazine. Regardless, Cope ignited the controversy that led to the work of both Bernard Fisher and his collaborators in the United States and Umberto Veronesi and his group in Italy.

In the 1970s Fisher and his colleagues began randomized controlled trials of the various surgical approaches to the treatment of women with a palpable, cancerous, small (2 cm or so) breast lump but no palpable lymph nodes in the axilla or evidence of metastatic disease elsewhere. One trial dealt with the aggressiveness of mastectomy. Another probed the relative effectiveness of breast-conserving surgery. In the former trial, one-third of the women received radical mastectomy, and one-third underwent simple mastectomy (only the breast is removed) followed by radiation therapy to the axilla. The other third underwent simple mastectomy alone, with a biopsy of the adjacent nodes. If that biopsy was positive for metastatic cancer, half underwent radical mastectomy and the other half had irradiation. The results of the twenty-five-year follow-up have been published. Women with negative lymph nodes had a 50 per cent likelihood of surviving for ten years without evidence of recurrent disease, while those with positive nodes had a 50 per cent likelihood of surviving only for five years without recurrence. Neither axillary radiation therapy nor more extensive surgery made a difference. These results at twenty-five years are commensurate with the results published in 1985 after ten years of follow-up. This earlier article turned medical heuristics upside down regarding the cure of breast cancer. It also inflamed the women's movement. Radical mastectomy, rather than heroic, turned out to be mutilating. There must be a gentler way to treat breast cancer, gentler even than simple mastectomy followed by armpit irradiation. Furthermore, given the survival differential favouring node-negative and, therefore, early detection of disease, wasn't there a way to find these tumours earlier, before they became palpable lumps? Both points were well taken, to say the least.

The first led to the demonstration that breast-conserving therapy served as well as simple mastectomy. In fact, in the US trial, lumpectomy was as effective in terms of survival from breast cancer as mastectomy, whether it was followed by irradiation or not. True, radiation therapy after lumpectomy reduces the local recurrence rate to that of simple mastectomy, but it does nothing for disease-free survival, the likelihood of distant metastases, or overall survival. It took twenty-five years for science to refute, incontrovertibly, "the more you cut, the more you cure" approach to treating this disease. No longer should any woman with a small breast cancer be offered mastectomy without due consideration of breast-conserving alternatives.

The second point – the more advanced the disease, the more likely it will kill the patient – is the rallying cry for early detection. It led to the flowering of mammography, and it continues to be a driving force today. Early detection, followed by a breast-conserving surgical and radiation therapy cure, is an accepted process. Certainly, such an approach holds more promise of cancer-free longevity than medical therapy of early or established disease. The evidence that we can "cure" metastatic breast cancer with non-surgical therapy, even today, is anything but compelling. In fact, the evidence that we can even prolong life demands scrutiny.

The oncology community publicizes its advancements, but the improvements are likely to be more apparent than real. Much of the "advance" can be ascribed to "lead-time bias," as our ability to detect metastases has steadily increased. The breast cancer that might have been deemed non-metastatic a decade ago can be shown to be metastatic today and labelled as such.

However, such cancer is more likely to have a natural history or progression approaching that of its "non-metastatic" than its "metastatic" forebear. We are foolish to think that the "improved" survival reflects effective treatment of metastatic disease rather than this difference in staging. Alvan Feinstein, the pioneering epidemiologist from Yale, called it the "Will Rogers Phenomenon," alluding to Rogers's Depression-era sarcasm that when the "Okies" left Oklahoma for California, they raised the mean IQ of both states. That aside, the literature on the effectiveness of variations in radiation therapy and chemotherapy following lumpectomy is as disappointing as it is extensive. It begs the refutationist treatment I am applying to all the topics in this book. Some of the most aggressive treatments, such as high-dose chemotherapy plus stem-cell transplants, have been shown to be useless, but only after thousands of women were subjected to them. Once women, and occasionally a man, start down this high-tech treatment path, they can only hope to be "survivors" of their breast cancer, rather than just survivors of the aggressive treatment that is today's heuristic.

For the well woman coming to grips with the spectre of breast cancer, the credo today is "early detection, hence early cure." That belief seems sensible, even incontrovertible. But there are provisos.

Proviso 1: Curing her breast cancer will not advantage all women

The ten-year and twenty-five-year data from the American trial comparing simple and radical mastectomy need to be examined closely. By ten years – or, actually, by five – the evil from breast cancer had largely played out. After ten years there was very little likelihood that any of the surviving women, node negative or positive, would experience recrudescence of breast cancer or die from it. But there was a very high likelihood that they would die of something else before the twenty-five years played out. The inception cohort was rich in women aged fifty to sixty-five years, and the average life expectancy for a woman who was sixty-five years old in 1979 was less than twenty years. The "something

Table 4.1
Incidences of Breast Cancer and of Death among Women over Their Life Span

Age	Still Alive	Incident Breast Cancers	Breast Cancer Deaths	Cardiovascular Deaths	Deaths from Other Causes
30–34	988	1	0	0	2
35–39	986	3	0	0	3
40–44	983	5	1	1	4
45–49	977	8	2	1	6
50–54	968	11	3	2	11
55–59	952	12	3	5	15
60–64	929	12	3	9	25
65–69	892	14	4	16	36
70–74	836	13	5	28	51
75–79	752	11	6	52	70
80–84	624	9	6	89	95
Over 85	434	5	7	224	203

else" they would die from includes all the other diseases vying for mortality primacy – the comorbidities, in epidemiology-speak. If you are approaching old age, or you are young but already burdened with diseases actively assaulting your longevity, breast cancer is less malignant a spectre and, in all probability, the least of your problems.

In an essay published in the *New England Journal of Medicine* in 2000, Kelly-Anne Phillips and her colleagues from Toronto made this point eloquently and reinforced it with the data based on a birth cohort of 1,000 Ontario girls. Table 4.1 presents their fate each five years over the course of their adult lives.

The first proviso appended to the credo of "early detection, hence early cure" relates to whether early cure will affect longevity or quality of life. It may be true, as the lay literature proclaims, that one in nine women will get breast cancer if they live to be eighty-five. Far fewer, however, will die from breast cancer or even know they have it when they die. Early detection, then, can advantage only those women whose breast cancer is a threat to their longevity. Early detection makes less sense as woman age or as they suffer more morbidities. In such circumstances, breast cancer is but one of the processes vying for the proximate cause of death, and not the most likely to win.

Based on the Fisher and Veronesi trials, however, women should not assume that the converse holds – that detecting tiny early cancers will necessarily advantage younger well women. The participants in these trials were selected because they had a palpable breast cancer but no palpable axillary adenopathy – enlarged lymph nodes in their armpit. This group is at high risk for death from breast cancer – 20 per cent of the women in the studies died from their cancer despite the various interventions. These are tragic losses, but we don't know whether one-fifth of the women with other presentations will suffer this same fate. We do know that both the self-examination and the clinical examination are highly unreliable and inefficient in detecting lumps, and that most lumps that are detected are not cancerous. Nonetheless, it is reasonable to postulate that the malignant potential would have been thwarted if the cancerous lumps in the 20 per cent who had fatal disease had been detected earlier and removed. But that does not mean that all lumps are as likely to metastasize or that all smaller breast cancers are likely to grow to palpable masses. We shall return to these thoughts in proviso 4.

Proviso 2: The course of breast cancer is not always inexorable

Our discussion of screening for colon cancer was facilitated by the predictable nature of colonic tumours, or neoplasia. The rate of transformation from polyp to metastatic cancer is still to be defined, but it is clearly both low in likelihood and slow in evolution. Polyps stay polyps for many years before they start to turn ugly. The same pertains to prostate cancer. Unfortunately, the story with breast cancer is not so straightforward. Women with palpable cancers are at greater risk of death from breast cancer, particularly those whose disease has metastasized to their axillary lymph nodes. But their fate is not sealed. As many as 40 per cent of women with positive axillary nodes survive ten years, and metastatic disease develops within ten years in 20 to 30 per cent of women with palpable breast cancers but negative nodes.

Breast cancer is a very heterogeneous disease. Probably, it's more than one disease. One subset behaves as though the

cancer is metastatic very early on, perhaps at the initial oncogenic events – the ones that altered the normal cell so that its
life-cycle and near neighbour interactions are cancerous. Some
breast cancers behave in similar ways to some lung cancers – as
though the oncogenic events occurred at multiple foci nearly
simultaneously. Unlike lung cancer, however, the clinical course
of the patient with metastatic breast disease can be extremely
unpredictable, sometimes seeming to find a stable plateau for
years before marching on. Some breast cancers have little malignant potential, certainly little that is relevant to the longevity of
most women. The breasts of a significant minority of elderly
woman harbour several such foci of cancer.

Proviso 3: Early detection may be illusive, if not ephemeral

The challenge is much more than the early detection of breast
cancer: rather, it is the early detection of breast cancer that
threatens the well-being and longevity of each particular woman.
This goal demands a screening tool that can detect cancers accurately and with such great sensitivity as to distinguish the more
potentially aggressive of the subsets that are still amenable to
surgery, or resection. The extent to which the screening instrument falls short in these characteristics is the extent to which
we subject well woman to anxiety and possible harm from treatment (iatrogenicity). The goal to screen so efficiently and effectively, however, may be unattainable. In that event, we must hope
for advances in science either to thwart the oncogenic event or
to redress the consequent pathobiology – to stop cells from turning cancerous or to learn how to cure cancers by turning off
unregulated growth in malignant cells.

To this day, mammography is the best screening tool we have,
but it is a blunt instrument. I doubt anyone would argue with
that assessment, though many might disagree with my opinion
that its use approaches travesty. Yet mammographic screening
has become an article of faith, a *cause célèbre*, and an industry for
various constituencies in the United States and some other
"advanced" countries.

To be useful, mammography must overcome two variables: the extraordinary variability in both the eyes of the observers and the radiodensity of normal breast tissue. A well woman must decide if mammography overcomes these variables sufficiently to attain the goal of sensible screening.

Radiologists vary, sometimes dramatically, when they read the same mammograms. In a study nearly a decade ago, a panel of ten radiologists read the same 150 mammograms, with no knowledge of the clinical course. For the mammograms from women who turned out to have cancer, the radiologists got the correct diagnosis between 74 per cent and 96 per cent of the time. For the mammograms from women who did not have the disease, cancer was highly suspected between 11 per cent and 65 per cent of the time. The false-negative rate is moderate and moderately variable. The false-positive rate is considerable and also quite variable. While training of mammographers has improved over the past decade, along with standardization of their machines and techniques, it is doubtful whether the reliability of readings among observers has become any better. More likely, it has led to increasing hesitancy on the part of the mammography community to read a mammogram as negative – a hesitancy that is fuelled by the fear of legal liability for false negative readings, but never for false positive readings. One prominent senior mammographer I am aware of informed a sixty-year-old patient that he would feel compelled to recommend biopsies every year, given the radiological appearance of her breast tissue. Rather than choose to eschew mammography, she chose bilateral simple mastectomies – and no cancer was found. The false-positive rate has escalated and, by the 1990s, over a third of women in screening programs had been faced with false positive results. That result translates into one negative biopsy per woman screened per decade.

Even if the interpretation of the mammographic image could be rendered reliable, screening would still be highly inaccurate. All radiographic images reflect the ability of the tissue to interfere with the passage of the x-rays to the detector. The more dense the tissue, the less the detector is exposed. The images are developed so that the denser the tissue, the more white the image. The image of a breast with a predominance of fatty tissue is black, allowing fibrous strands and glandular elements to stand out. Cancers, which are usually dense, sometimes with speculations, or white flecks, of calcified tissue, stand out on images of fatty breasts. However, fatty breasts are anything but the rule at any age. Younger women tend to have less fatty breasts, as the tissue is rich in glandular elements and their supporting connective tissue. Menopausal status, number of live births, post-menopausal estrogen therapy, and body mass index all influence breast density. Most important, breast density is a familial trait.

There is an increase in the risk for breast cancer in women with dense breasts – a risk that is not entirely a result of the compromise in mammographic sensitivity and one that may reflect the quantity of glandular tissue that can turn cancerous. The denser breast is therefore at greater risk for breast cancer – but, unfortunately, for a breast cancer that escapes detection by mammography. Considerable effort is under way to improve the sensitivity and specificity of mammography by using higher-resolution imaging techniques, some of which employ other processes such as ultrasound and MRI. Unfortunately, we are still waiting for compelling evidence of improvement in detection: the cancers remain nearly as furtive regardless of the technique. We seem to be asking more of this anatomical imaging technology than it can possibly deliver. Given the issues in reliability and accuracy, can mammography find the twelve new breast cancers that will occur in 929 women screened annually from the age sixty to sixty-four, as set out in table 4.1? All it will do is give the mammographers licence to recommend a biopsy in 150 of these women, including many of the twelve with breast cancer, but not necessarily the few whose cancer is life threatening.

Proviso 4: Not all breast cancers need to be detected

This proviso is a corollary to proviso 1 – not all breast cancers need to be cured. If nothing else, mammographic screening causes a lot of women to undergo a breast biopsy. The results are predictable, once you learn of the earlier experience with breast self-examination and clinical examination.

Early in the twentieth century, pathologists described small growths composed of the cell type that lines the ducts from the milk glands. The cells looked normal and did not seem to extend across the basement membrane that delineates the duct from the surrounding tissue. These small growths were thought to be "pre-cancers." By mid-century, labels such as "lobular carcinoma in situ" (LCIS) and "ductal carcinoma in situ" (DCIS) appeared in the literature. "Carcinoma" is another term for cancer, and "in situ" suggests that there is no discernible evidence for spread. No alarm was sounded. After all, these lesions were not palpable and were generally discovered incidentally in the proximity of benign nodules that were removed because they were palpable. With the growing emphasis on biopsying lesions discovered at self-examination, DCIS was a frequent incidental finding by the mid-1970s. At this same time, the notion of a "pre-cancer" really took hold. Surgeons writing in prestigious medical journals advocated mastectomy to expunge the risk, whatever its magnitude. Some went so far as to recommend random biopsies of the other breast, which, in 50 per cent of cases, revealed one or more foci of DCIS and, therefore, led to a recommendation of bilateral mastectomies. The "pre-cancer" notion evolved to denote one focus of DCIS as indicative of a predisposition to developing breast cancer. After all, as many as 70 per cent of breasts removed for a single lesion were found to have multiple foci of DCIS. If the label "pre-cancer" is allowed such weight, mastectomy seems sensible, particularly given the surgical hubris of the day.

DCIS may indeed be a "pre-cancer," but it is not a precursor to the palpable adenocarcinomas that were targeted in the Fisher and Veronesi trials. It can grow to be sizable, can be extensive (involving ducts out to the nipple, or Paget's disease), can be anaplastic (the cells can take on a more malignant appearance), and can be necrotic (the cells in the centre die, producing a "comedo carcinoma"). All these features are associated with increased recurrence at the site of excision if the DCIS is not completely excised. DCIS can also become invasive, and is more likely to be invasive if it has the features already mentioned. However, the low-grade, tiny DCIS lesions take their time to become invasive, and even more time for the subsequent invasive cancers to become metastatic. There is great uncertainty as to the timing of these transitions, but the conceptualization countenances decades. On this basis, as in colon cancer, a surgeon could justify excision in a younger patient.

We are witnessing an epidemic of DCIS. In 1980 DCIS accounted for only 2 per cent of breast cancers. Between 1973 and 1992, the age-adjusted incidence rate of DCIS increased nearly sixfold; the age-adjusted rise in the incidence of invasive ductal cancer was only 34 per cent. Women are not getting more cancers. Rather, US women are getting more breast biopsies thanks to mammography, and DCIS is the incidental finding of this exercise. However, DCIS is another New Age shibboleth; local excision is always recommended, often with some accompanying radiation therapy, with or without hormone therapy (usually tamoxifen). And local excision can be extensive – to assure both "clean margins" and an opting for painful and expensive breast reconstruction if total mastectomy is chosen.

I have grave doubts about this therapeutic posture. I suspect that little of importance, perhaps nothing, would be lost if all these women with tiny lesions, detected only on mammography, never knew they had DCIS. Lobular carcinoma in situ can be found in the breasts of as many as 18 per cent of women who die of unrelated causes. To me, this current approach is an exercise in circular reasoning. After all, you gain nothing for longevity by curing non-lethal lesions.

Proviso 5: Mammographic screening may be a social construction

Mammography, then, is a technique with compromised reliability, limited sensitivity, and troubling specificity. It is also a technique that results in an enormous number of negative breast biopsies. When it leads to a positive biopsy, it is far more likely to cause the extirpation of lesions that are best ignored, rather than being lethal, and it will miss many that are dangerous. In any screening test other than mammography, it would be relegated to the false-start category. But breast cancer is the prototype for Susan Sontag's *Illness as Metaphor* and is viewed as a plague. A "war" on breast cancer has become a crusade.

Mammography is not just blunt; it's so very blunt that it approaches being useless, and it's time we relegated it to the archives. That's not just a proclamation of a man of the academy. Three randomized controlled trials have tested whether mammography detects breast cancer in a way that advantages the women in the screening program – that increases the likelihood that something else will cause their death. None of these trials was American: one was Canadian, the other two were Swedish, and all three were sizable and lengthy. The Canadian randomized controlled trial tested whether adding mammography to an annual clinical breast examination improved any relevant outcome. The Stockholm and Malmö trials added screening mammography to usual care. There are at least four other scientific studies testing the same hypothesis, but they are less compelling because of less-powerful designs. These trials are of interest, but the randomized controlled trials supersede them.

The Canadian trial enrolled some 50,000 women aged forty to forty-nine and 39,000 women aged fifty to fifty-nine. The enrolment occurred between 1980 and 1985. All these women were examined at the inception of the cohort and received instruction on breast self-examination. They were randomized into two groups: one subjected to screening with annual mammography, and the other not so screened. There were three telling observations:

• After eleven to sixteen years of follow-up, 213 of the 50,000 women who were in their forties at inception of the cohort had died of breast cancer. These cancer deaths, and incident cancers that were not (yet) fatal, were distributed equally between the mammography group and the usual care group.

- After thirteen years of follow-up, of the 40,000 women who were in their fifties at inception of the cohort, 622 invasive and 71 in situ cancers had been detected in the group afforded mammography, compared to 610 and 16 in the group screened without mammography. There were 107 deaths from breast cancer among the women subjected to mammographic screening, and 105 among the women not so screened.
- Based on these data, several – but not all – august North American bodies have backed down from recommending mammographic screening in women in their forties. None has backed down from mammographic screening for women over the age of fifty. Several have waffled, including the US Preventive Services Task Force, which, in its 2002 report, recommends "screening mammography, with or without clinical breast examination, every 1 to 2 years for women aged 40 and older."

None of these professional bodies operates free of sociopolitical constraints. Two stouthearted participants published in the *Journal of the American Medical Association* the saga of the "consensus conference" convened by the National Institutes of Health in January 1997. The "consensus" was to equivocate on screening mammography in women in their forties. It was born in acrimony and it was met with acrimony. No only did the American Cancer Society disagree, but the US Senate passed a resolution repudiating the consensus, demanding revised guidelines, and convening investigative hearings. Steven Woolf and Robert Lawrence describe a climate and a response that was an assault on intellectual freedom. Three months after the consensus panel pontificated, the National Cancer Institute reversed its stand and recommended mammographic screening for women in their forties.

For those of us who support Karl Popper's refutationist ideas, this saga is dramatic but predictable. Many people, in many different constituencies, are committed to inculcating mammography into American life. It is the stand of the American news media in the 1990s, as documented by a published analysis of the coverage. Science is no match for such advocacy.

The science and its messengers are not viewed as refuting the hypothesis that screening mammography is a solution to the problem of woman dying of breast cancer. Rather, the messengers are viewed as callously refuting the problem itself. The messengers can be vilified, not just by those with vested and invested interests in promulgating mammography, but by the women on whose behalf the science is designed.

The Malmö trial enrolled 42,000 residents aged forty-five to seventy between 1976 and 1978. The Stockholm trials enrolled 60,000 residents in 1981. Both studies monitored their cohorts for at least eleven years. There was no suggestion that the women of Stockholm were spared death by breast cancer thanks to the mammography, though there was such a hint in the Malmö cohort. These trials have been reviewed and meta-analyzed many times and, because of methodological subtleties, the Stockholm trial is considered more lacking than the Malmö trial.

In 2001 two Danish investigators, Ole Olsen and Peter Gøtzsche, working under the impressive imprimatur of the Cochrane Collaboration (the international collaborative effort to offer "evidence-based" appraisals for many clinical challenges), published a series of articles examining the literature supporting the recommendations for screening mammography. Not surprisingly, they consider the Malmö and the Canadian trials as the only ones of sufficient quality to hold sway. Their interpretation is similar to mine: mammography offers very little, if anything, of value to the women screened. In addition, it causes the screened women to undergo a dramatic excess of surgical procedures and adjuvant therapies to no demonstrable avail.

There is a counter-argument, one based on a secondary analysis of the Malmö data and, therefore, inherently suspect. However, it comes from Olli Miettinen, a Finnish scholar, epidemiologist, and statistician who commands great respect in the world of epidemiology for his critical, inventive mind. He argues that older women, over the age of fifty-five, gained an important advantage thanks to mammography. Two decades after the screening, there was a 50 per cent decrease in deaths among women who had been screened compared to women who were never screened. To my mind, though, this outcome among a group of women who are all over the age of seventy-five hardly justifies all the screening, let alone all the unnecessary aggressive treatment.

Harold Sox, the editor of the *Annals of Internal Medicine*, has had a long-standing interest in evidence-based medicine, particularly in mammography. His comment on the US Preventive Services Task Force recommendations, and the state of the art in 2002, concluded with a mandate to keep women informed on the nuances of the debate. Suzanne Fletcher and Joan Elmore argue along the same lines for screening in women younger than fifty (whose close relatives have been spared breast or ovarian cancer early in life), although they still recommend screening for women aged fifty to sixty-nine. Steven Goodman, writing a companion editorial to Sox, points out how Swiftian the debate has become. If we take the most optimistic approach to these data as they relate to women in their forties, it is much ado about almost nothing of value. Much the same perspective applies to mammography in women fifty years of age or older.

5

Prostate Envy

The prostate is a walnut-sized gland that wraps itself around the male urethra as the urethra travels from the bladder towards the base of the penis. It is arguably more important for its role in disease than its function in health. After mid-life the normal prostate may grow in a disorganized fashion, so that the gland is filled with lumps, or nodules. The lumps that are benign, however, are exceedingly difficult to distinguish by palpation, or touch, from surrounding malignant changes. The time-honoured tradition of the "digital rectal exam" – to palpate the prostate for cancer – turns out to be as non-specific and insensitive as it is unpleasant and indelicate.

There is a strong probability that some of the cells in these benign nodules will lose their normal microscopic and biological features and take on the characteristics of cancerous cells. They will form a localized cluster of cancer cells, or carcinoma in situ. Nearly every man will have carcinoma in situ by the age of eighty, and probably most men by fifty. Obviously, the majority of men are never aware of the cancer they may harbour. These cells are generally slow to grow and slow to metastasize – to produce secondary tumours elsewhere in the body – so most men die from other causes long before their prostate cancer is ever symptomatic.

The biology of these cancer cells is different, including their propensity to secrete prostate-specific antigen (psa), a protein that normally remains largely in prostatic secretions. Because PSA is commonly measured in the blood, testing for this substance is frequently used in early detection programs. In general, the higher the level, the more likely the cancer is no longer hiding among the nodules. Persistent elevated numbers suggest that the cancer may have spread beyond the confines of the gland. But PSA measurement is a limited screening tool because it is not cancer specific. Normal prostate cells also secrete PSA, and inflammation and trauma can cause non-malignant prostate cells to secrete more of the antigen. Borderline PSA test results provide a reason to perform biopsies, and biopsies, in turn, often lead pathologists to incidentally find the cancerous cells lurking among the other glandular elements.

Once told that cancer has been found under the microscope, how many patients will turn away from the hope for a cure? Urologists recite probabilities based on PSA levels and the "Gleason score." This score is a measure of how invasive and distorted the cells appear under the microscope, though cancers that look to be extremely nasty are exceptional – and they may even represent a biologically distinctive form of the disease. Most carcinomas are not that distinctive when in situ, so most biopsies reveal little about the probability that the cancer will spread beyond the prostate gland.

In recent years, several well-known American men – Bob Dole, Arnold Palmer, Norman Schwarzkopf, Rudy Giuliani, and Colin Powell – have trumpeted their triumph over prostate cancer. All learned of their diagnosis thanks to PSA screening. All suffered through the subsequent investigations: the prostate biopsies, blood tests, and imaging studies that proved they had prostate cancer but determined it was still confined to the gland. They met the enemy and vanquished it. "Victory" came via a surgical procedure, the radical prostatectomy, which is designed to remove the entire gland but spare the urethra and nerves that course through the region. These nerves are responsible in part for bladder control and erectile function. All four men bear scars of the battle, and some have more than surgical scars. Dole, for one, can be seen on television advertising the pharmaceutical he takes to treat his erectile dysfunction. These men claim that engaging this enemy was tactically sound: they feel brave in their battling, and they justify any untoward consequences by the assurance that death by prostate cancer will not be their fate. They say they have won this war on cancer.

Each year in the United States some 200,000 men learn they are affected by prostate cancer. Half will choose the cure promised by removing their prostates; others will choose less invasive procedures involving radiation therapy, either from an external source or from radioactive pellets implanted into the prostate. These non-surgical procedures are obviously less invasive, but, over time, they may also be less certain to eradicate the cancer. The less invasive treatments are less likely to result in erectile dysfunction and urinary incontinence. Spouses, peers, and the public at large applaud men who incisively confront their cancer. They have overcome anxiety, risked indignity and pain, and subjugated morbidity in order to reap this benefit of modern medicine. Their triumph lights the path so others will follow. They are heroes of the war on cancer, marching arm in arm with the predominantly female survivors of breast cancer.

Most physicians recommend PSA screening for prostate cancer. If the screening is negative, the patient sighs in relief. If the screening is positive, the enemy is revealed – with luck, in time to combat it successfully. Screening awareness is everywhere, from the daily press to a stamp issued by the US postal service which called for "Prostate Cancer Awareness: Annual Checkups and Tests." William Catalona of Washington University and Patrick Walsh of Johns Hopkins Hospital are two urologists who have attained near celebrity status as proponents of screening and the algorithm, or decision path, it engenders, particularly the one that leads to radical prostatectomy. Not surprisingly, the American Urological Association recommends screening. Urologists and the hospitals in which they practise advertise "screening days" as a public service.

American men expect to be screened. Any physician who advises otherwise has much to explain and may well be ripe for

Table 5.1
Mortality Results in the Scandinavian Trial

	Watchful Waiting	Prostatectomy	Relative Hazard (%)
Deaths from prostate cancer	31	16	50
Overall mortality	62	53	83

a malpractice suit. Prostate screening is seen as a right of passage and makes sense. There's only one problem: it doesn't work.

THE SCANDINAVIAN TRIAL

The futility of prostate screening is obvious from the results of several randomized controlled trials that have been published. The first, from Scandinavia, appeared in the *New England Journal of Medicine* in the fall of 2002.

In 1988 a group of Scandinavian investigators began recruiting healthy men under the age of seventy-five who had untreated and newly diagnosed prostate cancers. The tumour had to be at an early stage: confined to the prostate, secreting limited levels of PSA into the blood, and meeting certain criteria in appearance under the microscope. Most prostate cancer detected by PSA screening would fit these conditions. By 1999 a total of 695 men were registered in the study. As they enrolled, the volunteers were randomly divided into two groups: half underwent a radical prostatectomy, and the other half were assigned to a period of "watchful waiting" under medical supervision. By 2000 the participants had been followed for an average of six years. The critical results are set out in table 5.1.

Because men of different ages entered the cohort at different times, the analysis of these outcomes requires careful statistical consideration. Some men were followed longer than others, and some were older and less likely to survive to 2000 even if they didn't have prostate cancer. Table 5.1 demonstrates that if the volunteer was assigned to undergo radical prostatectomy, he was 50 per cent less likely to die of prostate cancer. But he was as likely to be dead by the year 2000 from some other cause (the

relative hazard of 83 per cent was too likely to occur by chance
for the 17 per cent reduction in hazard to be meaningful).*
Prostatectomy does not change the date of death; all it changes
is the likelihood that prostate cancer will be the direct cause.

There's another daunting message in table 5.1. True, the men
treated by "watchful waiting" were twice as likely to die of prostate cancer, but those who underwent the procedure were not
spared that fate. Six years after radical prostatectomy, 16 of the
347 men died of prostate cancer – a crude mortality rate of
5 per cent. Even though their disease was defined as being in
an "early" stage, it wasn't; or perhaps the "radical" prostatectomy
was not radical enough. Regardless, no man should think that
surgery is guaranteed to vanquish his risk of death from prostate
cancer; it will reduce it at best by only a half. And no man should
think that surgery will increase his time on earth; all it will
change is the likelihood of the mode of demise, the proximate
cause of death.

The Scandinavian study also probed the personal cost of radical prostatectomy. The sexual, urinary, and bowel functions of
the volunteers were monitored, along with certain other aspects

---

*Throughout this book the reader will come across terms such as
odds ratio, hazard ratio, relative risk, and *relative hazard,* as well as
terms such as *risk reduction* and *hazard reduction.* They are all statistical constructs. The various ratios are not synonymous, but they are
close. I am using them in their formal sense, but the reader can
treat them as synonymous. However, they demand close attention
if one is to discern the degree to which they are meaningful. In
the example in table 5.1, the chance of dying from prostate cancer is reduced from 31 per cent to 16 per cent by radical prostatectomy – a 50 per cent reduction in the hazard of death from
prostate cancer. If it were reduced from 2 per cent to 1 per cent,
that too would be a 50 per cent reduction in the hazard of death
from prostate cancer. Such a small effect probably cannot be measured reliably, but even if it were a reliable reduction, few men
would choose the procedure, given the tradeoffs in table 5.2.

Table 5.2
Erectile and Urinary Function Results in the Scandinavian Trial (per cent)

Function	Prostatectomy	Watchful Waiting
ERECTILE FUNCTION		
Greatly distressful dysfunction	30	17
Greatly distressful decreased intercourse	28	16
URINARY LEAKAGE		
Moderately or greatly distressed by	29	9
Regular dependence on diaper or bag	14	1

of their quality of life. Table 5.2 sets out the notable results in this personal area of investigation.

Because the volunteers made up an elderly and aging cohort, members of the "watchful waiting" group were not spared other urological disorders. In fact, they suffered more from obstructive symptoms than the prostatectomy group. As the aging male prostate enlarges, it's common for multiple benign nodules to impinge on the urethra as it passes through the gland. This "benign prostatic hypertrophy" (BPH) is a normal part of the aging process and is the cause of prostatism – increased urinary frequency, decreased forcefulness of the urinary stream, and dribbling. Transurethral prostatectomy (TURP) is a limited surgical procedure that removes only the impinging nodules, with improvement in prostatism. Radical prostatectomy removes the entire prostate, nodules and all, which also decreases the likelihood of prostatism. However, nearly 15 per cent of the patients who undergo radical prostatectomy will have incontinence problems and be obliged to wear a diaper. Almost as many will be afflicted with erectile dysfunction because of the surgery. For most men, these consequences are catastrophic.

Interestingly, there was no discernible difference between the two groups in the Swedish study in overall physical and psychological functioning. Nearly half of all these aging men described themselves as suffering decreased physical capacity, a moderate or high degree of worry, and a low or moderate personal quality of life. The result was the same whether they were subjected to radical prostatectomy or they were just observed. Once they were identified with prostate cancer, it seems, they viewed themselves as patients, rather than healthy men, and the burdens of urinary incontinence and erectile dysfunction were subsumed under this pall.

Why does an otherwise well man opt for screening for prostate cancer? If the digital rectal exam or the PSA is positive, and then the biopsy is positive, the radical prostatectomy he may choose to undergo might provide a 50 per cent decrease in the likelihood that he will die of prostate cancer. The procedure will, however, make little or no change in the timing of his death or the overall quality of his life. In 15 per cent of patients, it is also likely to produce a major problem with erectile and urinary function. Given these facts, prostatectomy is not, in my opinion, a reasonable choice, nor are gentler options that have a similar benefit/risk ratio. The drug finasteride, for example, which inhibits a patient's ability to produce active androgens, the male sex hormones, has a small preventive effect on the formation of nodules in the prostate. If this drug proves to be effective in helping to reduce the incidence of prostate cancer, the tradeoff will be that the men who still go on to develop prostate cancer will suffer a more aggressive form. To me, that's not a defensible gamble.

THE PROSTATES OF SEATTLE V. THE PROSTATES OF CONNECTICUT

The 1990s witnessed the flowering of the PSA screening agenda, but its implementation was not uniform across the United States. The Medicare beneficiaries aged sixty-five to seventy-nine residing in the Seattle area between 1987 and 1997 were five times more likely to be screened, and twice as likely to be biopsied than the Medicare cohort residing in Connecticut. It follows that the Seattle cohort was more likely to be "helped" by early treatment of cancers. Nearly 3 per cent of the Seattle cohort underwent radical prostatectomy, and another 4 per cent had radiation therapy. The respective numbers in Connecticut were 0.5 per cent and 3 per cent. However, there was no difference between the two groups in the likelihood of dying from prostate cancer. In fact, there was no difference in prostate-specific cancer mortality if the patients were biopsied in any of three age group-ings in that span. Yet these are the ages at which nearly all pros-tate-specific deaths occur. Death from prostate cancer before the age of sixty-five is much less common.

The Seattle-Connecticut comparison is an observational, or "ecological," cohort study. As such, it is not as powerful a test as the randomized controlled trial on the utility of PSA screening. Nonetheless, the take-home messages of both this study and the Scandinavian experiment are consistent.

PSA SCREENING IS DISAPPOINTING AT BEST AND PROBABLY HARMFUL

In one British survey of patients with suspected or confirmed prostate cancer, few men knew that the benefit from screening was so tenuous. Those who became aware of this evidence regretted having been tested. Screening can be meddlesome: it turns healthy men with positive tests into patients, with no demonstrable improvement in the end result. Perhaps the risk/benefit ratio would be compelling if radical prostatectomy were reserved for the rare individuals whose PSA and Gleason scores were both extremely high and who still had no evidence of meta-static spread beyond the prostate. That is a hypothesis ripe for testing. I wouldn't be surprised to learn, however, that the sur-gery does not advantage even this subset. It is possible that such tumours spread very early, rendering any surgery "after the fact."

The literature relating to screening for prostate cancer is voluminous, contentious, and difficult. The American Academy of Family Physicians advises counselling men over fifty; the American Cancer Society recommends annual PSA testing for men over that same age; the American College of Physicians recommends individual decision making; the American Medi-cal Association calls mass screening "premature"; the Canadian Task Force on Preventive Health Care found "fair evidence" for screening; and Medicare includes annual screening as a standard benefit.

Given the mixed messages from these medical associations, I am writing this book in the hope of arming readers with the "hard" questions to ask before they submit to any screening program for prostate cancer.

PART TWO
Worried Sick

The Last Well Person is the one who is able to confront clinical science without being medicalized and to harness it for personal benefit. I have written this book to prepare the reader for this task.

Part One lays out the clinical science that is relevant to our mortality. That exercise forced us to shed a number of pre-suppositions, particularly the idea that mortality is an abstraction, a formless beast we can bring to heel by the determined application of the latest and most convincing insights. Our forefathers were frequently seduced by the pronouncements of the sages, particularly the religious sages, about the path to a good, if not a longer, life. Today we wait for the next pronouncements of the biomedical establishment.

Readers of this book have seen, however, that longevity is anything but abstract. The death rate is one per person, and the time of death is set near our eighty-fifth birthday. Any claim to a science that offers a path to longevity beyond this age is fatuous. The challenge for each of us is to recognize that science has uncovered ways to increase the likelihood that we will arrive at our eighty-fifth birthday feeling reasonably well, even healthful, regardless of our burden of disease. We care little about how many diseases we have or which of our diseases causes our death, so long as we can readily cope with the challenges our diseases present and, when our time comes, our passing is swift. Clinical science, including its newly born biotechnology, has something to contribute to our quest for longevity thus defined, but not much. After all, three-quarters of our mortal hazard resides in the social structure of the course of our lives, as reflected in our socioeconomic status and kindred measures. Science has been nibbling at the other quarter for years, claiming great success of late and marketing its presumed prowess. Part One largely puts this dialectic to rest, even though a grain or two of value can be found among the chaff. The Last Well Person is a match for the claims of modern science regarding longevity.

Part Two addresses this crucial issue of coping with life's challenges. It is the secret to being the Last Well Person. To be well is not to be free of physical and emotional symptoms and problems. If that were the definition of "well," there would never be a well person, at least not one who was well for long. Life, normal life and its living, is replete with intermittent and remittent morbidity. To be well is to be able to cope efficiently and effectively with the challenges.

Hans-Georg Gadamer lived into old age and earned his place in the pantheon of twentieth-century philosophers. Gadamer held medicine in the highest regard when it stared into "the face of illness ... to discover the great enigma of health." He realized that to be well was not simply to be free of disease: "The fundamental fact remains that it is illness and not health which 'objectifies' itself, which confronts us as something opposed to us and which forces itself on us ... The real mystery lies in the hidden character of health. Health does not actually present itself to us. Of course one can also attempt to establish standard values for health. But the attempt to impose these standard values on a healthy individual would only result in making that person ill. It lies in the nature of health that it sustains its own proper balance and proportion. The appeal to standard values which are derived by averaging out different empirical data and then simply applied to particular cases is inappropriate to determining health and cannot be forced upon it." The discussion of the metabolic syndrome in chapter 2 illustrates the way in which the imposing of "standard values on a healthy individual" results in labelling many people as ill, thereby medicalizing "healthy individuals" so that they grasp at unproven remedies for contrived diseases that are said to be life threatening.

Gadamer first penned his observation into the enigma of health in 1991. By then there was a literature – or science, if you prefer – that could have informed this insight. However, it resided in the margins of the clinical and epidemiological literatures, corners seldom visited by philosophers of the day. In 1991 that literature was scant; today it is the product of a mature science. These writings will inform our discussion in this second part and will be detailed in the annotated readings. They attempt to define and quantify health, in contrast to the traditional epidemiological literature, which attempts to define and quantify illness. The traditional literature takes the patient as its reference point. The epidemiology of health takes the experience of morbidity in community-dwelling people as its reference point. It is the scientific analysis of well-being.

The assertion that coping with intermittent and remittent morbidities is "normal" is on firm scientific grounds. None of us will live long without headache, backache, heartache, heartburn, diarrhea, constipation, sadness, malaise, or other symptoms of some kind. When we pause in recognition of any such morbid challenge, we are faced with a predicament. For my purposes, "predicament" is a convenient term because it captures the challenge without casting aspersions or assuming causation. We all have personal predicaments that often challenge our sense of well-being. Some are catastrophic: overwhelming chest or abdominal pain, acute neurological symptoms, broken bones, and the like. For these events, choosing to be a patient of someone licensed to practise medicine or surgery is more than sensible – it's mandatory. Modern medicine has much to offer if we fall victim to such events: it provides cures for some and important comfort for others. Most personal predicaments are less catastrophic morbid events, but they are still disconcerting. Because they are less than catastrophic, we have the opportunity to pause and consider what to do. Some predicaments have been medicalized to such good effect that it is as sensible to seek medical care for them as it is for the catastrophic events – burning on urination, fever and a productive cough, abnormal vaginal bleeding, for example. However, for many other personal predicaments, the appropriate recourse is less certain or even contentious. We will explore several such predicaments that are bound to colour our lives at some time. There is a science that elucidates our choosing among the options, and everyone must choose. For the Last Well Person, the choosing will be informed.

One choice is to "deal with it" – to cope in our own way. If we choose to do so, we will remain a person with a predicament for as long as the morbidity persists. We will all take recourse in our common sense. Common sense is a reflection of our own previous experience and the notions of those we listen to. Even without giving voice to our predicament, we will not feel isolated. From every side – family members, the lay press, purveyors of sundries – we will hear of options in conceptualizing the predicament and in palliation. Are these suggestions salutary? How are we to know? How will we fare as a person with a predicament?

We can, of course, choose to seek care. For most personal predicaments, there is a menu of options in providers of care. Each of the options proclaims a theoretical underpinning, uses a privileged language, offers a peculiar treatment act, and provides an assortment of procedures by people with specialized training. These professionals have been admitted to their practice after submitting to review by their peers. Some submit to ongoing peer review, and some maintain the privilege of their practice through licence. If we choose to avail ourselves of one of these options, we will no longer be a person with a predicament. We will be a patient or a client with an illness or a condition – and, likely, forever. We will learn the language and conceptualizations of the professional into whose hands we have consigned ourselves. Our self-image will change, as will our idioms of distress and of wellness. We will be different.

The pressure to choose any option or any particular option reflects our common sense, just as choosing to remain a person with a predicament does too. If we choose to seek the care of someone licensed to practise medicine or surgery, we change from a person with a predicament to a patient with an illness. This particular transition is termed "medicalization." Medicalization has a pejorative connotation, which is appropriate if we are not better off for the choice. Before choosing to be a patient of a physician or a chiropractor, or the client of a herbalist, physical therapist, or other purveyor, the Last Well Person will consider the ramifications and decide whether that option will be advantageous.

Part Two is a discussion of predicaments and these options. As with Part One, I am choosing predicaments and options that are exemplary but not inclusive. Many more topics are worthy of similar treatment. Sorely missing from this part, for example, are discussions of the predicaments of heartache and heartburn. The former goes by terms such as depression and affective disorders; the latter by waterbrash, dyspepsia, and gastroesophageal reflux disease (GERD). "Sinusitis" and allergies also deserve critical appraisal. However, I have space limitations – and there will be another day.

6

Musculoskeletal Predicaments

Regional musculoskeletal disorders are symptoms that afflict working-age people who are otherwise well, who have no complicating major neurological deficits, and who have suffered no violent or even specific cause. A region of their musculoskeletal system hurts, particularly when that part is used. Most episodes of backache, neck pain, knee pain, shoulder pain, and the like are regional musculoskeletal disorders – and they are common. They rank second as the reason anyone seeks primary medical care, and first as the reason workers suffer long-term disability. They are the *raison d'être* for entire professions such as the chiropractic, osteopathy, and manual therapies. They have left an indelible mark on language, in terms such as "ruptured disc" or "tennis elbow." And suppositions about the regional musculo-skeletal disorders – their cause and their cure – are a powerful contemporary social construction.

Regional musculoskeletal disorders support a great number of people in myriad therapeutic facilities. Pharmaceutical laboratories and a variety of factories produce a wide range of supposedly palliative pills and devices to help those in pain. Burgeoning bureaucracies contend with sources of funding to support all this activity, while various public and private indemnity schemes provide recourse for those whose pain is insurmountable. Given this investment by so many different partners, it's no wonder that the conventional treatment for regional musculoskeletal disorders

has withstood the science that finds their social construction
fatally flawed and even harmful.

This branch of medicine has witnessed some of the most dramatic, real-time, and relevant clinical advances in the past fifty
years, all of which challenge the very being of a large clinical
establishment and a powerful insurance industry. These breakthroughs may be making slow inroads into the behaviour of both
the medical fraternity and health insurance, but they have barely
a foothold in the community. Given the predictable lag time, the
Last Well Person must learn to be proactive.

Here are ten state-of-the-science tenets – Popperian "truths"
yet to be disproved – about regional musculoskeletal disorders.
All have been largely ignored by society and by the medical and
insurance institutions that are meant to serve us. These tenets
demand close attention if any one of us is to fend for ourselves
or stave off harmful notions and interventions.

- The regional musculoskeletal disorders are intermittent and
  remittent predicaments of life. It is distinctly abnormal to live
  two years without an important backache, or three years without important neck and arm pain, or five years without important knee pain. By important, I mean pain that lasts weeks,
  even months, and causes us to alter our customary life activities
  – in other words, pain that is memorable.
- Less important episodes are far more common, more fleeting,
  and less memorable, but still notable predicaments when we
  have them. If we were to keep a diary of every morbid aspect
  of each day for six weeks, well over half of us would have
  something to record. The most common morbidity relates to
  upper respiratory symptoms though half of us would record
  regional musculoskeletal pain, most frequently low-back pain
  that is likely to last one week out of the six. Few, however,
  would feel the need to make more than minor alterations in
  lifestyle.
- The majority of us manage with these predicaments without
  seeking care from medical or other providers. That holds for
  both the fleeting and the prolonged episodes. Most of us

manage to cope so effectively that the episode is not even memorable. How we cope varies from person to person and place to place, according to previous experiences and cultural presuppositions. For example, the consumption of non-opiate analgesics, pain-killing pharmaceuticals over the counter and by prescription, can be enhanced by clever marketing, even though science can discern little effectiveness or any difference in benefit or in the likelihood of toxicity in all of them. The tendency for people to consume "neutriceuticals" such as chondroitin and glucosamine is driven mostly by rumours circulated in lay publications. Compounds of this nature can be sold without scientific or regulatory scrutiny, and some individuals, it seems, will always cast about for offbeat remedies.

• Previous experiences and cultural presuppositions also play their part in influencing some people to seek professional assistance in coping. This choice is determined by a far more powerful force than marketing. If your life is not in order, the regional musculoskeletal disorder will seem more severe and the need for professional care more pressing. Family discord, psychosocial stresses, financial insecurity, and job dissatisfactions are prime movers in this regard. The particular health-care provider individuals choose reflects their own previous experiences, the reports from others they know, and marketing by the providers themselves. But the need to choose a provider is driven by psychosocial confounders that impede the ability of people to cope on their own.

• In choosing to be a patient with a regional musculoskeletal disorder, clients are, in truth, voicing a surrogate complaint. The presenting complaint may be "My back (or shoulder, or knee) hurts," but those words are surrogate for "My back (or shoulder, or knee) hurts, and I can't cope with this episode." If that was the stated complaint, or the complaint inferred by the provider, interventions could be fashioned that address both the painful anatomy and the compromised coping. Addressing just the first symptom is inadequate.

• When workers find their back or arm pain disabling, the content of their tasks is seldom as limiting as the negative context in which they labour (as we will see in chapter 9). For the elderly woman with knee pain, the limiting lesion is far more likely to be psychosocial – often loneliness – than anatomical.

- It is normal to have degenerative changes of the musculo-skeletal system. If you have a pristine spine at mid-life, that is distinctly "abnormal." Our ability to define which abnormality is the cause of a particular episode of axial pain (backache or neck pain) is small – too small to justify any imaging study. It isn't much better for "pinched nerve," the radicular (nerve root) pain that shoots down the arm or leg (sciatica). Whatever we see on the magnetic resonance image (MRI) is likely to have been present before the individual started to hurt and will likely persist when the person heals. The discal hypothesis – the idea promulgated seventy years ago that the "ruptured disc" is the culprit – has not withstood scientific scrutiny well. It is largely untenable for axial pain, and marginal for radicular pain. Most asymptomatic adults have impressive discal pathology by the age of fifty, as do all who manage to make it to eighty-five. Regardless of whether this discal pathology occurred suddenly or was painful, it caused no particularly memorable predicament. "Ruptured disc" and "bad back" are terms that deserve to be relegated to the historical archives.

- Knee pain is another intermittent and remittent predicament of life. Memorable knee pain will afflict up to 20 per cent of us each year, whether we are twenty years old or seventy. As with the axial skeleton, the episodes of pain are nearly totally discordant from any demonstrable anatomical abnormality at all ages. Most knee joints that hurt have no demonstrable pathology, and most with demonstrable pathology don't hurt. That holds for damaged menisci, cruciate ligaments, and cartilage surfaces. We have learned that the knees of persons whose lifestyles incorporate considerable weight bearing are more likely to have better cartilage as well as spur formation (osteophytes), one of the classical changes of osteoarthritis. It seems there are "good" and "bad" spurs, good spurs forming around healthy, well-used joints, and bad spurs forming around joints that are suffering the loss of cartilage and biomechanical integrity we call osteoarthritis.

- The common denominator of the myriad interventions purveyed as specific treatments for regional disorders is lack of effectiveness. There are more than two hundred randomized controlled trials of treatments for axial pain, yet none of the various forms of poking, prodding, injecting, exercising, yanking, girding, needling, and the like can be shown to consistently and robustly offer any advantage over placebo events. None of the pharmaceuticals has effectiveness, efficacy, risk/benefit ratios, or cost/benefit ratios that exceed that of low doses of aspirin or acetaminophen. There is not even a hint that surgery for regional axial pain is helpful. There is a hint that surgery for radicular pain might help some. Total hip replacement is a solution to biomechanical compromise, the abnormality in hip motion, as well as hip pain. But there is no suggestion that surgery for knee pain is similarly helpful. Reconstruction for knee instability may help with gait, but knee pain is a tenuous indication. So, too, for shoulder, elbow, and wrist pain. Surgery for nearly all regional musculoskeletal pain has earned its place in the historical archives next to tonsillectomies, hysterectomies for retroverted uteruses, radical mastectomies, and other misguided empiricisms. Unfortunately, surgery for the regional musculoskeletal disorders has become an industry.

- We do not know what causes particular episodes of regional musculoskeletal pain. The risk from specific tasks on or off the job is trivial, so we have no more reason to label a regional backache an injury than we have to label a spontaneous headache an injury. The motion that causes the back to hurt is unlikely to be the motion that caused the discomfort in the first place. Labelling lateral elbow pain "tennis elbow," even if you don't play tennis, should sound the nonsense it is. That term is no more sensible than calling angina the "stair climber's chest." The state of the science is such that when a person complains of regional knee pain, the most valid

diagnosis is likely "a painful knee" – and the same pattern
holds for regional shoulder pain, back pain, and neck pain.
Some day, maybe soon, we will have a handle on the micro-
anatomy and biochemistry that is at play, and that understanding will suggest new diagnostic labels whose validity is
worthy of testing. But the traditional labels that imply pathoanatomy or causation are no longer tenable.

These ten tenets can arm us to cope with our next episode of
regional musculoskeletal pain, and they are well supported by
the literature. I will now present five circumstances of regional
musculoskeletal pain – circumstances that each of us is likely to
suffer during our lives, and ones that demonstrate how a person
informed by these tenets might cope.

A prototypical episode of acute regional backache   It started mid-
morning when you bent over to tie your shoelace. Suddenly there
was searing pain, low in the back, and you could barely stand
up. It has settled slightly since onset, though you still can't
stand erect. You can walk, listing, with great difficulty, and sitting
at your desk offers some relief. Aside from the difficulty of getting to the bathroom, bowel and bladder function are intact.
You have no lower extremity symptoms – no weakness or loss of
sensation. You're just miserably uncomfortable, particularly
when you move. You recognize your plight as an acute backache,
just as you might recognize you had the "flu." You are not alarmed,
but you are disconcerted that, for the next few days, if not weeks,
discomfort will compromise your normal activities. That will take
some understanding on the part of your family, employer, and
co-workers. There has been some friction at work, but your boss
should be willing to accommodate you if you are diplomatic in
your approach. Perhaps that business trip could be postponed
and you could focus on deskwork instead. The acetaminophen
you took an hour ago is taking the edge off. You'll remember to
repeat that dosage a few times a day. Several house chores can
also be postponed and your spouse can empathize, having had

a similar episode last year. You'll make the best of it and get on with life. This too shall pass.

Subacute regional shoulder pain   The discomfort has been insidiously getting worse for a week now. At this point, reaching behind to fasten a brassiere is too painful to accomplish. Brushing your hair with the right hand is impossible. Fortunately, there are front-fastening bras to circumvent the first disability, and the left hand to circumvent the second. That does not make this circumstance any less disconcerting. It's particularly annoying at night: rolling over onto the right shoulder can awaken you with pain. You are no match for your weekly tennis game. The good news is that, aside from compromise in reach, dexterity is preserved. The bad news is that you know such regional shoulder pain often takes months to run its course. You might as well hunker down for this longer haul. Acetaminophen and a warm shower at bedtime help get you through the night, most nights. Your fitness should not suffer if you switch to jogging or another aerobic lower-extremity routine, though your tennis game might. You bemoan the fact that modern medicine is no match for this predicament. Doctors might demonstrate some anatomical abnormality at the right shoulder, perhaps of the rotator cuff, but there is a high likelihood that they'd find the same pathology at the other cuff. So who knows what's really hurting? Maybe a steroid shot would help; maybe not. Certainly there is no surgical solution, not even an arthroscopic solution. It's annoying, to say the least. But this too shall pass.

Regional knee pain at the age of twenty-five   You're a fit, recreational athlete – at least you thought so until the past month. First intermittently and now more persistently, your left knee hurts. It seems a bit swollen and feels tight. You tried jogging but didn't get far before the knee felt unstable and caused you to limp. You paid a price for the next few days with increased swelling, discomfort, and limping. You have a friend who had a similar experience last year. He saw Dr Jones, a local orthopaedist, who organized an MRI of the knee, followed by arthroscopy to remove a torn meniscus and then several months of physical therapy and progressive exercises. Only now is your friend back to speed. You're tempted to pursue the same recourse, particularly since your health insurance will pay nearly all the fees. But you read *The Last Well Person* and learned that all the studies show your friend would have recovered even sooner had he let the knee heal spontaneously. You also became aware of the long-term data on damage to the knee associated with open meniscectomy, "the answer" twenty years ago. More recent data on the "less-invasive" arthroscopic meniscectomy is pointing in the same direction. You opt for spontaneous healing and, to maintain the muscular tone of your leg that is essential for normal knee function, you alter your fitness regimen to avoid activities that have an undue impact on the knee. Cycling for a couple of months sounds reasonable, maybe swimming a little. This too shall pass.

Regional knee pain at the age of fifty-five   Maybe it was the abuse from playing football in high school, although you don't remember any severe injuries. You have been a recreational jogger since college, but that's no explanation; there are studies of people like you and they fare better than most. Although you're fit, you have episodes of nagging left knee pain when you limp, you are cautious in descending stairs, and you are faced with a stiff knee when you wake in the mornings. Your knee feels tight and unstable and, although it has never given way, you feel too insecure to jog or play tennis. You worry that you're following the same path as your father, who, by the time he was your age, was hobbled by bad knees. At least, today, a total knee replacement might save you from that fate. But isn't there something to do short of that? Arthroscopic surgery is no longer an option, not since the randomized controlled trial published in the *New England Journal of Medicine* suggested you would be worse off for that effort. You decide against the glucosamine/chondroitin sulfate treatment because the data that these products are useful is marginal, particularly since the purveyors underwrote the more positive studies. You'll just have to figure out some way to make the best of your condition. Non-weight-bearing sports like cycling and swimming will become the mainstay of your fitness regimen. And you'll try to keep slim so you will burden the knee as little as possible when it's hurting. This may not pass, but if the pain does not progress, that's good enough.

Chronic neck pain with radiculopathy at the age of sixty   For months you've had a nagging pain in your neck that comes and goes. You have to be careful backing out of the driveway, since your neck won't rotate sufficiently to see over your shoulder. Sleeping is difficult, too: you can find a comfortable position and fall asleep, but one turn and you're up and hurting. Recently this annoying neck pain was joined by a pain that ran down the outside of the right arm towards the wrist, along with numbness, tingling, and some loss of sensation in the middle fingers. You coped with the neck pain, but this arm symptom, or radiculopathy, was too uncomfortable and disconcerting to tackle alone.

Your family doctor referred you to a neurosurgeon, who found your physical examination reassuring in that there was no weakness, though she did note the loss of a reflex in your arm. After you underwent an MRI, she explained that there was a lot of degenerative disease, including spurs and disc space narrowing, at multiple levels and on both sides of your neck. Although she couldn't be certain as to which abnormality was pinching the nerve provoking the arm symptoms, the radiculopathy pointed to the problem being at or near a particular nerve root. She offered you surgery, both to remove any spur or the like from the neighbourhood of that root and to "stabilize" that region of the neck with hardware so it couldn't move and pinch the nerve again.

You thanked the neurosurgeon but demurred. You were aware that this surgical approach was based on a theory that had never been tested. The neurosurgeon was extrapolating from flawed studies for radiculopathy at the low back (sciatica). Those studies suggested that the radiculopathy responded somewhat to the surgery, although the natural history lagged by only a couple of months – not a good enough reason for you to submit to surgery. As long as the neurological symptoms did not progress, you would take your chances that the condition would heal on its own. You were not even tempted to try a neck collar or accept a referral to physical therapy. Soft neck collars do little more than remind you to sit erect so you don't unduly stress whatever is hurting by flexing your neck forward. You have adjusted the height of your computer and the like to accomplish as much. And studies have shown that physical and manual therapists have little effective to offer. You'll trust the natural history, even though you may have residual symptoms for months to come.

Are these five vignettes contrived? If you ask members of the treating professions, most would doubt that there are many people in the United States who could cope with these predicaments in this fashion. It takes more than self-assurance; it requires empathy, support, and encouragement from family, friends, co-workers, employers, and the community. Without such support, it takes extraordinary fortitude and certitude to withstand the advice of neighbours who view themselves as beneficiaries (survivors) of modern treatments, as well as the pronouncements of a phalanx of professional practitioners in purchased advertisements and in the lay press. However, community-based epidemiology suggests that many people do cope in this fashion – perhaps the majority of those with these particular predicaments. Furthermore, they do so by relying much more on their personal and community resources than on having any comprehensive grasp of the relevant science that supports their approach. Those who seek professional assistance in coping are more likely to lack a supportive community, or they are seduced by the purveyors of help and the people who think they were beneficiaries of such help. If you are faced with the predicament of a regional musculoskeletal disorder, there are only a few sensible reasons for abandoning your personhood for the patient-client role, and no sensible reasons for abandoning you control over your fate.

- If you are not comfortable with your assessment that you are suffering from a regional disorder, you should seek reassurance from an appropriately trained professional. That means if you feel poorly, have fevers, or are losing weight, or if the pain is not clearly "mechanical" – relieved by rest and exacerbated by usage – or if you have important neurological symptoms such as weakness in a limb or difficulty with bladder or bowel function. Otherwise, it is sensible to remain a person and try to cope till your predicament resolves itself.

- If you are comfortable that your predicament is a regional disorder, but there seem to be insurmountable barriers to coping, then, perhaps, you should seek assistance from an astute professional. Be prepared to engage in a discourse about psychosocial influences that might be the critical confounders. Discussions of troubles in life at home or at work should not be taken as irrelevant or offensive, because problems of this kind are responsible for impairing your ability to cope with the pain. Airing these concerns is sensible.

- If you do succumb to the promises of treatment, at least be certain that you will benefit from the concepts you are expected to assimilate and the procedures you are offered. If you are comfortable talking about pressure points, unstable segments, discal herniations, subluxations, vital forces, and other similar fallacies, then go ahead. If you find comfort in being stretched, poked, girded, injected, arthroscoped, or even fused, so be it. That is your choice. I would hope, however, that you are paying for these treatments out of pocket and not through health insurance. If you want to participate in a therapeutic paralogism, you should pay for it yourself. I don't want to share the expense by virtue of the magnitude of my health insurance premiums or my taxes.

Such is the state of the science today. The changes I am suggesting have serious ramifications for many insurance schemes. The regional musculoskeletal disorders are the rubric under which much of the expense in workers' compensation and other disability indemnity is cost-accounted. In most industrialized countries, workers' compensation insurance is a federal benefit, often funded from general tax revenues. In the United

States, however, fifty-eight different jurisdictions regulate these indemnity schemes, most of which mandate that employers provide insurance themselves or purchase it from private sector purveyors. Whatever the system, the number of claims and the cost incurred has been an issue since the mid-twentieth century, escalating dramatically since the 1980s largely because of disabling regional low-back pain and the other regional musculoskeletal disorders. Furthermore, the claims are rising in spite of interventions, mainly in the area of ergonomics.

In 1983 the Quebec Workers' Health and Safety Commission established the Quebec Task Force on Spinal Disorders to examine this trend. The commission asked the task force to explain, for example, why the escalation had not been blunted by the continual increase in physiotherapy treatments in Quebec, which had risen to 641,197 in 1982. To this end, Dr Walter O. Spitzer, chairman of the Department of Clinical Epidemiology at McGill University, assembled representatives from many of the relevant clinical disciplines and charged them with performing one of the first systematic reviews of the scientific literature on the diagnosis and treatment of neck and low-back regional disorders. The group considered well-done randomized controlled trials the most persuasive. They gave little weight to uncontrolled but structured descriptive studies and literature reviews, and dismissed all anecdotal reports. Of some 4,000 studies they considered, they rated 469 as informative. To the alarm of the industrialized world, they found that almost nothing in the diagnostic and therapeutic armamentarium was on firm scientific footing. Several procedures and interventions had been shown to be useless or even harmful. Their report stood as a reproach to the relevant professions, a clarion call for science of higher quality and reform of the approach to medical indemnity.

The Quebec document still remains a model for similar exercises in other fields, as well as for updated exercises for regional musculoskeletal disorders. The most influential of the updates was initiated by the US Department of Health and Human Services nearly a decade later, when Congress funded the Agency for Health Care Policy and Research to examine the effectiveness and cost-effectiveness of health care delivered under the Medicare program, a national health insurance scheme for retired and disabled workers. A panel constituted under Dr Stanley Bigos was charged with developing an evidence-based Clinical Practice Guideline for "acute low-back problems in adults." Members of this group (on which I served as a consultant) considered another 4,000 articles, published after the Quebec review, and they deemed about 10 per cent of them to be informative. Two years later the published guideline reached conclusions very similar to those of the Quebec Task Force. In the years since, nearly every industrialized country has concurred with this report, often after establishing an investigatory task force of its own. New Zealand's 1999 report specifically addressed diagnostic and therapeutic issues that relate to the psychosocial confounders to coping.

It is possible that great progress is just around the corner. After all, people with musculoskeletal disorders are living with painful and limiting predicaments for which no anatomical explanation holds up to scrutiny. Perhaps a different, more fertile explanation, likely at the biochemical level, will some day be found. Many new agents in development are worthy of testing, and a vast market awaits any such success. Many a drug will be touted as effective, and some will gain the approval of the FDA. The recent history of the development and introduction of the COXIBS – the latest in the long line of analgesic and anti-inflammatory drugs seeking to supplant aspirin in the medicine chest – is an object lesson in why the Last Well Person should be sophisticated about the process and wary of the hype that too often masquerades as "progress." The origins of this story go back a long way.

THE COXIB CANARD

The first multinational pharmaceutical firm was the Jesuit order. "Peruvian bark," the miracle drug of the seventeenth century, was also known as "Jesuit bark" because it was harvested from the chincona tree by indigenous South Americans and imported by the Jesuits. This "Jesuit tea" was an antipyretic, an agent that could reduce the fevers and agues that plagued Europeans, and it was quite effective, since the active ingredient was quinine. Though Western physicians had no remedy that compared favourably with Jesuit tea, they held it in great disdain. They were therefore receptive when the Rev. Edward Stone wrote to the Royal Society of Medicine in London in 1763 that the bark of the willow tree, the "sallow" tree of the species *Salix*, had similar properties to Peruvian bark. This "battle of the barks," which played out till the close of the nineteenth century, was the first skirmish of the nonsteroidal anti-inflammatory drug (NSAID) wars.

That same century end also saw the flowering of Prussian organic chemistry. The active principle of willow bark was isolated, labelled salicin, and chemically modified to produce a number of congeners (chemically related substances), some of which were found to be pharmacologically active. In this pre-drug trial era, effectiveness was literally judged by observation, and toxicity was easily overlooked. At the turn of the twentieth century, salicylic acid was used to "burn" warts, while sodium salicylate was a widely used antipyretic despite the fact that it induced nausea more frequently than potions based on quinine. Other salicylates remained on chemists' shelves. Acetyl salicylic acid had been synthesized in pure form in 1869 and labelled aspirin ("a" for acetyl and "spir" for the Spirsäure plant from which the salicylic acid was isolated). It remained on the shelf of the I.G. Farbenfabriken in Bayer-Eberfeld until Felix Hofmann, a chemist, treated his father with that compound for arthritis. The Western world would never be the same again.

At that time, Friedrich Carl Duisberg Jr was a young chemist with Friedrich Bayer & Co., a minor player in the dye chemistry industry. He understood that chemistry could produce more than industrial compounds, including products that would supplant biologicals in the pharmacopoeia and in medicine chests around the world. Aspirin was a natural, since the market was vast and his company its leading manufacturer. In 1903 Duisberg travelled to Rensselaer, New York, and built a factory. He was the marketing genius who emblazoned the "Bayer Cross" on many more products than pills and transformed the company into the enormous industrial powerhouse known as I.G. Farbenindustrie AG – I.G. Farben. The Rensselaer factory came under American ownership during the First World War, sold to a patent medicine firm that evolved into Sterling Products. Sterling purveyed "Bayer aspirin" until a decade ago, when corporate reshuffling returned the name and the brand to German shores. In the meantime, aspirin had found a huge market around the world, including the developing world. Bristol-Myers, American Home, and Miles Laboratories joined Sterling in competing among themselves and with I.G. Farben for the sale of aspirin and preparations containing aspirin. Sales grew unchallenged until the 1960s, when tons of these pills were consumed each day in the United States alone.

In the 1930s another product of nineteenth-century Prussian chemists, long collecting dust, started a tortuous journey to commercial success. It emerged in force in the 1950s into the British market and then into the United States as acetaminophen, which was marketed as Tylenol by McNeil Pharmaceuticals. When Johnson & Johnson, an enormous purveyor of consumer health products, purchased McNeil, Tylenol competed directly with Datril, the Bristol-Myers version. Both made important inroads into the aspirin market as an analgesic and antipyretic. Although acetaminophen has little of aspirin's effect on the swelling, redness, and warmth that characterizes inflammatory lesions, it does not cause epigastric burning or intestinal bleeding. This advantage positioned it well in the battle with aspirin.

In mid-century, Boots, the venerable British retail drug chain, added a small research division to its company to try to develop a new anti-inflammatory agent as powerful as corticosteroids (steroids) but without the toxicities of steroids or aspirin. Stewart Adams, a young pharmacologist, and John Nicholson, a biochemist, were lucky and discovered a new NSAID, ibuprofen, which was patented in the late 1960s and marketed shortly thereafter as Brufen in Britain and as Motrin, under licence to Upjohn, in the United States. The floodgates to NSAID development and the vicious marketing it engendered had opened.

Motrin was the first anti-inflammatory agent to undergo scrutiny by the modern Food and Drug Administration (FDA), the agency charged with testing both the safety and the efficacy of drugs before they can be released for public consumption. Under this regime, every approved NSAID has been shown to be more effective than a placebo; no approved NSAID has been shown to be less effective than aspirin; no approved NSAID has been shown to be more effective than aspirin; and no approved NSAID has been shown to be safer than aspirin.

There is one more element of the story to outline before we tackle the COXIB debacle. Generations of scientists have sought the mechanism by which aspirin is anti-inflammatory. Many theories have proven untenable, but one has stood the test of time and clearly explains some, and maybe most, of the action. In 1971 Sir John Vane, working for Burroughs-Wellcome in Britain, discovered that aspirin (and all NSAIDs) inhibited the enzyme cyclooxygenase (COX), which is critical in the biosynthesis of prostaglandins, known mediators of inflammation. Vane was awarded a Nobel Prize for this insight. Prostaglandins are also involved in maintaining the integrity of the stomach lining, so that inhibition explains the NSAID gastropathy – the shallow erosions that come and go in everyone who ingests NSAIDs. In the early 1990s it was shown that there were two forms of COX: COX-1, which is present in many cells, and COX-2, which could be induced in certain cells. Experimental studies suggested that COX-1 was active both in inflammatory processes and in the stomach, whereas COX-2 was more exclusive to inflammatory processes. The race was on for a new NSAID that inhibited only COX-2 – an effective anti-inflammatory agent that spared the stomach, or, in other words, the perfect aspirin. Several such compounds were discovered in the laboratories of several pharmaceutical firms, much to the profit of their stockholders. These new NSAIDs were called COXIBs, to denote that they were specific COX-2 cyclooxygenase inhibitors. Two, now marketed as Celebrex and Vioxx, were the first to be tested in trials and to pass muster with the FDA.

The trials recruited patients with either rheumatoid arthritis or regional musculoskeletal disorders – usually knee pain in the setting of osteoarthritis. These demanding and expensive trials are increasingly outsourced to contracted research organizations (CROS), private sector enterprises that service the pharmaceutical industry by managing the clinical trials, the data analysis, and the application process before the FDA. CROS, or another specialized contracted organization, recruit physicians, who in turn recruit subjects from their practices. The CROS, the physicians, and, usually, the patients all receive remuneration for their participation. Long gone are the days when drug trials were free of vested interests, conflicts of interest, marketing undercurrents, and fraud. Some scandals involving "paper patients" and data massaging have been noted in the national press and have forced regulatory agencies to monitor the quality of the trials. The COXIB example is among the more subtle ones.

The Pharmacia and Merck pharmaceutical companies sponsor numerous professional symposia and dinner talks by "thought leaders," and they advertise both in professional journals and directly to consumers. Spending on direct-to-consumer advertising of prescription drugs by the pharmaceutical industry tripled between 1996 and 2000 to $2.5 billion (which is only 15 per cent of the total pharmaceutical marketing budget). The yield can be equally impressive. Celebrex and Vioxx each accounts for revenues that exceed $3 billion per year. Merck and Pharmacia have convinced consumers and prescribers that their COXIBS are worth the considerable extra expense compared to inexpensive over-the-counter aspirin and other NSAIDS. The advertising campaigns suggest that a sufferer can enjoy relief with diminished risk of gastrointestinal toxicity, as was predicted by the test-tube studies of the COX-2 inhibitors. Despite these claims, neither company has ever generated data that convinced the FDA (or me). One has to question why the FDA licensed COXIBS in the first place, given that the agency was not convinced of any advance in effectiveness or in safety over available drugs with long-term track records.

Once licensed, the enormous success of the new cox-2 agents provides testimony to the power of rumour, the gullibility of the lay press, and a slick approach to marketing to both physicians and patients. For example, shortly after Celebrex was released, Jerome Groopman wrote a glowing article in the *New Yorker* that relied on attestations of the principal scientist of Pharmacia's pharmaceutical subsidiary that developed the agent. Groopman was writing as a medical journalist. The influence of physicians who are writing or speaking as "experts" can be more insidious if their interests, and the interests of patients, are in conflict to any degree. For example, when the American College of Rheumatology convened a "subcommittee" to "update" the "recommendations for the medical management of osteoarthritis of the hip and knee," the guidelines argued that the risk/benefit ratio favoured coxibs for patients over sixty-five years of age. Yet, when the four members of the subcommittee were asked to disclose their "relationships" – such as paid consultancies or speaking contracts – with pharmaceutical or biotechnology companies, they listed four, nine, eleven, and seventeen such arrangements, respectively, mainly to companies in the NSAID business and with COXIB producers as the common denominator. The Last Well Person should realize that this example is no longer an exception in the United States.

In spite of the exorbitant profits, neither Pharmacia or Merck, nor their stockholders, was content in sharing the market. Both companies sponsored large clinical trials attempting to demonstrate safety to the satisfaction of the FDA, so that the "serious gastrointestinal toxicity" forewarning could be expunged from the labelling and the marketing materials. Pharmacia's CLASS trial appeared in the *Journal of the American Medical Association* (*JAMA*) in 2000, comparing Celebrex with ibuprofen or diclofenac (Voltaren) in patients with rheumatoid arthritis and with regional musculoskeletal pain in the setting of osteoarthritis (mostly regional knee pain). Merck's VIGOR trial appeared in the *New England Journal of Medicine*. It compared Vioxx with naproxen in rheumatoid arthritis. So armed, the pharmaceutical firms and their hired CROs petitioned the FDA to expunge the warning.

Neither the FDA's in-house reviewers nor its advisory panel was convinced by the CLASS trial data. When the statistical analysis offered by Pharmacia was scrutinized, there was no demonstrable advantage to Celebrex. However, the FDA's reviewers and the advisory panel differed on whether there was a discernible margin of gastrointestinal safety when Vioxx was compared with naproxen. The FDA's in-house reviewers were not impressed, but the advisory panel thought there might be an edge, though not one sufficient to assume an advantage over all NSAIDs. Merck's victory proved Pyrrhic. An unanticipated finding of the VIGOR trial was apparent to both groups of reviewers: there were more cardiovascular deaths in the patients on Vioxx than on naproxen. Is this result a statistical fluke? Or is it a toxicity of all COXIBs that was not apparent in the CLASS trial because low-dose aspirin was allowed?

Alternatively, is there nothing about the CLASS trial that is credible? When investigative reporters learned that the CLASS trial had been published with incomplete data, they publicized the story widely. The completed data that was presented to the FDA later contradicted the published conclusions. The FDA reviewers were correct in their conclusion that Celebrex offered no risk/benefit advantage whatsoever. It was later learned that the complete data was available at the time the paper was submitted, but that someone decided to publish the incomplete data and its analysis, which appeared to favour Celebrex. Subsequent marketing was based on this publication: 30,000 reprints of the *JAMA* article were purchased for distribution. Celebrex sales increased from $2.6 billion in 2000 to $3.1 billion in 2001. The CLASS trial masthead listed sixteen authors: six were employees of Pharmacia, and the rest had academic affiliations but were paid consultants for Pharmacia – the funder for the study. One of the academic affiliated authors had a long-standing financial relationship with Pharmacia and other drug firms, was the lead author of an earlier Celebrex trial, and currently directs the division of the FDA responsible for reviewing anti-inflammatory new drug applications.

Sidney Wolfe, who leads the Health Research Group of the advocacy organization Public Citizen, is serving the public as watchdog over the FDA's drug licensing process. It is unfortunate that we need a watchdog, for there is a sensible alternative. It's time to take the testing of drugs out of the private sector. We could establish federally funded "clinimetrics" units at selected medical schools, staffed by appropriately trained investigators who would be prohibited from establishing fiscal relationships with pharmaceutical companies. The companies would still patent their drugs, test them in animal models, and carry out the early phases of clinical testing. But the industry would no longer perform the definitive randomized controlled trials. A panel of clinimetricians would prioritize new drugs for trial based on the likelihood of an important advance. In an article I published in 1983, I suggested a biostatistical methodology that would take advantage of enrolling a limited number of patients in each of a limited number of testing sites. "Me too" and "minor effect" drugs would disappear rapidly and cheaply in this process, as would much of the vested interest. So, too, would the CRO and related industries. Unfortunately, much is vested in perpetuating the current approach.

Meanwhile, the marketing of Celebrex and Vioxx continues, joined by Bextra and others. There is so much at stake, and so much money in play, that the marketing minions have marshalled forces that are a match for this FDA setback following the CLASS and VIGOR trials. An alarming number of physicians, including academicians, have assumed paid roles in the process of performing clinical trials and marketing drugs. Some trials are designed to be marketing exercises rather than attempts to test hypotheses as to risk/benefit ratios. An alarming number of publications are written and lectures delivered by individuals with pharmaceutical company income, just as a huge number of articles describing trials are authored by physicians who had no direct control over the design or data analysis, and who take to the hustings in sponsored lectures, workshops, and publications. None of these practices has escaped attention, but the behaviours continue unabated.

The most disconcerting aspect of the COXIB example is that the entire enterprise is based on a misconception. NSAID gastropathy comes and goes while patients are on these agents; it is totally discordant from symptoms, and it bodes no evil in most people. NSAIDs increase the likelihood of important gastrointestinal complications in very small, easily defined subpopulations: those with a previous history of ulcers, those on ulcerogenic drugs (such as steroids and alcohol), those who are taking anticoagulants (blood thinners), those with a prior history of clinically important ulcer complications, and the elderly – particularly women. For the rest of us, NSAIDs are no hazard. For the subsets at risk, the sensible advice is to avoid exposure and to prescribe acetaminophen – the first-line alternative analgesic. COXIBs, for this group, are simply not an option.

Overall, the marketing of NSAIDs over the past forty years has been very effective. Some 80 per cent of US adults report taking over-the-counter analgesics frequently during the course of a year – some very frequently. Physicians in the United States wrote more than 312 million prescriptions for analgesics in the year 2000, and 140 million prescriptions for narcotics in 2002. Talk about medicalization!

7

Medicalization of the "Worried Well"

Someday I hope to hear that a Westerner stood before a Western physician and said, "Doc, I feel awful. Could it be in my mind?" And that the physician replied, "I hope so. That's a lot better than leukemia, or renal failure, or lupus, or the like."

For most Westerners, especially for most North Americans, such repartee is anathema. It is tantamount to an admission of whining or feigning or just being "crazy." A recent study from Edinburgh confirms that most Westerners are offended by suggestions that their symptoms are in their mind. New patients attending a general neurology outpatient clinic were interviewed before they saw the doctor. The patients were asked, "How would you respond if you had leg weakness, your tests were normal, and a doctor said you had X?" Table 7.1 is culled from this study, with some liberty. I am using less vernacular responses – the connotation "putting it on" is tabulated as "feigning," for example. For each presumptive diagnosis, the percentage of patients who impute a negative connotation is tabulated. The authors went on to compute the "number needed to offend," based on the idea that people are most offended if they think they are being accused all at once of malingering, of confabulating, and of being crazy. Telling patients their symptoms are "in your mind" will offend 50 per cent to this degree. "In your mind" will offend about a third of the patients with any of the next four labels to this degree. About 10–20 per cent with the next three labels are

Table 7.1
Edinburgh Study of Connotations of Medical Diagnosis (per cent)

Diagnosis	Feigning	Crazy	Imagining
Symptoms all in your mind	83	31	87
Hysterical weakness	45	24	45
Psychosomatic weakness	24	12	20
Medically unexplained weakness	24	12	31
Depression-associated weakness	21	7	20
Stress-related weakness	9	6	14
Chronic fatigue	9	2	10
Functional weakness	7	2	8
Stroke	2	5	5
Multiple sclerosis	0	1	3

so offended. A small number are offended if the diagnosis is "stroke," and even fewer by a diagnosis of multiple sclerosis.

This study is an exercise in semiotics. The investigation is probing the symbolism in these labels. Hysterical weakness, psychosomatic weakness, depression-associated weakness, and stress-related weakness are not as offensive as "all in your mind," though all these terms imply that the symptom is perceptual rather than a reflection of end-organ pathology. They, like "functional weakness," are essentially synonymous with "in your mind," but carry little such baggage. Overtly declaring uncertainty with the diagnosis of "medically unexplained weakness" is heard as more offensive than a label of uncertain clinical value, "chronic fatigue," which has cachet in the public mind. Clearly, the establishment of rapport in the medical treatment act plays out within well-circumscribed semantic boundaries, which reflect the culture of the day. Someone with physical complaints, such as regional musculoskeletal pain, carries definite preconceived expectations into the treatment act. People do not seek the ministrations of a physician to hear magical thinking, such as invocation of some vitalistic force, to explain symptoms. Nor do they want to hear from a physician that their symptoms are perceptual in nature. Rather, they seek out a physician to learn the "scientific" cause of the symptoms, with the expectation that the cause will be remedied and that the symptoms will regress.

This presumption has not always been so. Michel Foucault, in his elegant monograph *The Birth of the Clinic*, dates this conception of the contemporary treatment act to the turn of the eighteenth century. Earlier, symptoms were considered to be diseases. Fever was a disease, along with agues, rheumatism, lumbago, catarrh, and other conditions. If you sought medical care because you were coughing up phlegm (sputum), you would be treated for catarrh – for coughing up phlegm. Unctions, potions, and worse would be plied, along with pontifications as to prognosis. Some generations of physicians have produced an iconoclast or two who can bludgeon the prevailing dogma until it yields to progress. In the early eighteenth century in London, Thomas Sydenham realized the fallacy of this diagnostic reasoning and posited that symptoms were the illness; in other words, the illness is the presenting manifestation of an underlying causal disorder, a disease. This insight was a major intellectual achievement, truly a paradigm shift from illness as disease to illness as an indication of disease. Without it we would still be treating catarrh instead of pneumonia, rheumatism instead of rheumatic fever, and so on. Without Sydenham's insight, scourges such as smallpox and polio would not be history. Modern medicine is anchored on this illness-disease paradigm and rightfully rejoices in its many successes. Westerners seek medical care expecting to be cured, and Americans demand it. Lynn Payer says it well in her monograph *Medicine & Culture*: "The American regards himself as naturally healthy. It therefore stands to reason that if he becomes ill, there must be a cause for the illness, preferably one that comes from without and can be quickly dealt with ... Such a system gives primacy to the idea that disease is some wild and hairy monster that can be locked up with diagnosis." Unfortunately, this success has a downside.

The illness-disease paradigm has enjoyed nearly three hundred years of acceptance and is firmly embedded in our culture. To question its essence is not just heresy; it is irrational. However, to assume that this paradigm is without shortcomings is ignorance. What do we do when the disease that underlies the illness remains indeterminate, despite modern diagnostics? What about the possibility of suffering illness in the absence of disease? Would the illness then qualify as a medicalization of a life event?

The disease is indeterminate Despite an ancient tradition that decries hubris, the admission "I don't know" is not a regular feature of many treatment acts. The doctor's uncertainty is often camouflaged by the differential diagnosis or as a "syndrome" diagnosis, which is nothing more than a New Age categorization of symptoms. The former has the virtue of structuring the clinical investigations; the latter of providing some basis for prognostication. My only qualm about such obeisance to hubris rises when the labelling is not comforting to the patient.

I'm troubled, however, when the "don't know" admission is banished, and not just hidden, by an unproved and usually self-serving clinical heuristic. Proclamations beginning with the phrase "in my experience" or "it is common practice" often take iatrogenic licence with the illness-disease paradigm. This practice has left indelible and inexcusable marks on the history of medicine. It can be a form of quackery that masquerades as science and usually operates as follows. Given the belief that there must be a disease underlying every illness, it is seductive to assume that any demonstrable coincident abnormality, or difference, is the likely culprit. The twentieth century witnessed the removal of countless tonsils to protect children from pharyngitis and of many retroverted uteruses for backache before prescient judgment, and then the appropriate epidemiological studies, took hold. It took a generation of observers before it was clear that children outgrow recurrent pharyngitis with or without tonsillectomy. It took two generations of observers before it was clear that retroverted uteruses are normal and present in a significant minority of perfectly well women (usually the angle at the juncture of the cervix with the uterus points the uterus towards the front; in 15 per cent of women, however, the juncture angles back towards the spine, so the uterus is retroverted). Many medically similar examples remain in practice today – some in use without the backing of any scientific testing, and some in direct contravention of science. Part One of this monograph bears witness.

Illness without disease   Payer's observation that Americans regard themselves as naturally healthy is telling. For that to be true, we Americans must be convinced of our invincibility. As we have seen in previous chapters, however, life presents us with morbid challenges. Our sense of invincibility is repeatedly under attack. Take the example of regional musculoskeletal disorders, the episodes of pain and restricted function that target discrete anatomical regions in people who are otherwise well and who have suffered no unusual precipitant. If questioned closely, nearly all of us can recall low-back pain in the last year. A third of us can recall pain at the shoulder, and nearly as many can recall pain at the hand, elbow, or wrist that lasted at least a week. Regional musculoskeletal pain is but one of the intermittent and remittent predicaments of normal life. Feeling "well" demands the sense of invincibility that we can cope with our next musculoskeletal or other symptoms. Being "well" means that we had the wherewithal to cope with the last challenge so effectively that it is barely a memory, if at all. It does not mean avoiding these challenges, for heartache, heartburn, headache, and all the other aches are part of life.

I emphasize regional musculoskeletal disorders here because they are the chief complaint of a sizable minority of people who seek the ministrations of primary care physicians and of the vast majority who consult chiropractors and other practitioners of manual medicine. It has long been accepted as common sense that a press towards recourse, to potions or the helping professions, is driven by the physical intensity of the person's predicament. The more severe the pain, the more it is memorable, the more likely the person is to consume analgesics, to experience work incapacity, and to seek professional care. Epidemiology has put this common sense to the test and found it is not tenable. Any compromise in the person's wherewithal to cope with regional musculoskeletal disorder supersedes both the severity of the pain and any compromise in function in driving our response.

This insight has important implications for the clinical treatment act. The narrative of distress of a patient with a regional musculoskeletal disorder is often delivered as a substitute for difficulties the person is having in coping with the demands of life that render the musculoskeletal disorder the last straw. "My back hurts" may well mean "My back hurts, but I'm here because I can't cope with this episode," or, more particularly, "... because I can't cope with this episode as well as the turmoil at home (or work)." Yet treatment acts for back pain are wont to focus exclusively on the back. The same can be said of treatment acts for shoulder pain focusing on the shoulder, knee pain on the knee, and so on. Such is the patient's expectation in seeking care, and the expertise purveyed by the chosen professional. The clinical contract demands specific treatment for the cause of the pain. Yet for nearly all the regional musculoskeletal disorders, such a treatment act rests on the shakiest of scientific grounds. It follows as no surprise that the response of these patients to primary care and other treatment acts cannot be shown to facilitate remission, though several of the treatments may render the patient less dissatisfied with the pace of the natural history. Perhaps this ineffectiveness reflects the inability to design specific treatment for discrete disorders. For back pain, more than three hundred randomized controlled trials have tested pharmaceuticals, advice about activity, a variety of gadgets, and many physical "modalities" – all without a hint of benefit (except for some slight improvement from a single osteopathic back crack administered after two weeks to patients whose illness is not confounded by sociopolitical factors such as work incapacity). I suspect these treatment acts don't work because they focus on the pathoanatomy, and not the psychosocial confounders to coping. To resort to cliché, they miss the forest for the trees. Regardless of the fact that these treatment acts do not work, the patient is instructed on the various clinical hypotheses on which the treatments are based. Needless to say, such instruction will irretrievably alter the patient's conception of his own health, as well as the general choice of idioms to describe current and future distress.

Persistent widespread pain   Hidden in all the community surveys of people with discrete regional musculoskeletal disorders are individuals burdened with persistent pain at multiple sites. Their numbers are impressive, varying between 3 and 10 per cent of the population, depending on the definition used and the community studied, but only recently has their plight been recognized. People with regional musculoskeletal pain at multiple sites are more likely to manifest psychological disturbance and to report other physical, or somatic, symptoms than people who suffer from, or recall, discrete regional disorders. They are frequent consumers of medical care. These individuals are often bedevilled by so many life challenges that any quest for some sense of being well, let alone of invincibility, is doomed. The intermittent and remittent morbid predicaments of life that well people find surmountable are insufferable and unforgettable setbacks for those living under this pall. Hence, they take note of and report other somatic symptoms. Variation in bowel habits looms large, and diminished vigour oppresses them. *Joie de vivre* is absent.

I suspect that few people suffering with persistent chronic pain suffer in silence. I further suspect that their narrative of distress depends on the listener. The idioms of distress that enlist the empathy of a clergyman are not the same as those that enhance communication with a social worker, a sibling, or a physician. We have no data on how these unhappy people select a confidant, but their cultural setting is likely to influence this decision. If they are seduced by the blandishment of "scientific" or pseudo-scientific medicine, they will choose a physician or some other health practitioner. As we have seen, the medical contract demands specific treatment for the cause of the pain, though the treatment provided, seemingly rational or not, is unlikely to have a scientific grounding. Such supposedly scientific treatment acts abound, generally predicated on a circularity of argument. The symptoms are ranked, a specific pathology is postulated, and a neologic diagnostic label is applied that reiterates the presenting symptoms. This labelling exercise is but "catarrh" redux. All the while, the treatment act is plying the patient with intimations about the pathophysiology of the painfulness.

This sequence of events shows how individuals suffering persistent widespread pain learn to be patients with "fibromyalgia." The clinician can find no specific cause for the complaint of persistent widespread pain but feels compelled to discern that the patient dislikes being poked at particular bodily sites. Since fibromyalgia is defined as a state of chronic widespread pain and tenderness at certain points, the clinician pronounces, "You have fibromyalgia." Any clinician who applies the fibromyalgia label and promulgates a treatment act on that basis must disregard the observation that putatively diagnostic "tender points" are related to generalized pain and pain behaviour. Fibromyalgia denotes nothing more than persistent widespread pain. However, in the labelling, the patient is forever changed. As the patient learns more about fibromyalgia, her narrative becomes laced with the new knowledge, which is then recited with an objectivity that approaches the dispassionate.

The fate of patients with persistent widespread pain labelled as fibromyalgia stands in reproach to whatever theory underpins this labelling and the subsequent treatment acts. In the community, the majority of people with persistent widespread pain improve with time, but those labelled with fibromyalgia seldom do. Based on the science that pertains to the regional musculoskeletal disorders, I suggest that this unhappy fate is not solely a reflection of the intensity of their symptoms or the pervasiveness of the psychosocial factors that confounded their coping so they chose to be patients in the first place. Rather, the treatment acts, saddled with empty promises of elucidation and unproved promises of palliation, are in themselves harmful, or iatrogenic. These circular treatment acts will only exacerbate whatever mood or thought disorder is complicating the plight of the patients.

The proponents of the fibromyalgia construction are convinced that their pathophysiological insights and theories are valid, though as yet unproved, and their therapeutic approaches need but tweaking to produce the benefits that have eluded demonstration to date. They could, of course, be right, but, undoubtedly, their approach is causing harm today. I admit it is

possible that a therapeutic triumph is but one scientific discovery away, rendering my psychosocial and sociocultural synthesis
secondary, if not fatuous. After all, it would not have been far
fetched to have constructed sociocultural models for the pathogenesis of pulmonary tuberculosis and AIDS were it not for the
superseding microbiology. Many an intrepid investigator has
stalked the cause of fibromyalgia in the labyrinth of our neuro-
endocrine and immune systems for just that reason, but clues
are hard to come by, and subtle changes prove unreliable, secondary, or non-specific. We now know that genetics plays little,
if any, role: none emerged from an analysis of eleven-year-old
Finnish twins and their families, 10 per cent of whom suffered
persistent widespread pain. Other investigators have sought
associations with unusual psychological or physical traumatic
events, but the results are inconsistent at best. Testing biomedical theories is proving difficult but not insurmountable. To
date, no such theories have survived formal testing.

Life under a pall   My psychosocial and sociocultural theory has
not survived formal testing either, and, indeed, such testing is
difficult to design and perform. I am suggesting that chronic
persistent pain is an ideation, or somatization, engendered in
response to the living of life under a pall, and not vice versa. I
am not defining "pall" further because my theory countenances
a wide range of individual differences in this tendency to somatize. These unfortunate people choose to be patients because
they have exhausted their wherewithal to cope. If this suggestion
is correct, the complaint of persistent widespread pain should
initiate a treatment act quite different from that leading to labelling as fibromyalgia. The symptoms of persistent widespread
pain should be heard as probable surrogate complaints for difficulties in coping with life's sometimes overwhelming problems.
Months, often years, of poking, testing, pharmaceutical products, and medicalization might be avoided by directly approaching the coping challenge. Patients should be spared instruction
in illness behaviours or in contending with contrived neolo-
gisms, such as "central sensitization," which connotes little more

than illness in the mind. Then they would avoid having to unlearn illness behaviours with "cognitive behaviour therapy" or the like.

There is no more valid a diagnostic label for patients complaining of persistent widespread pain than "overwhelming persistent widespread pain." Certainly, fibromyalgia means nothing more. Leading investigators are promulgating two other labels: "functional somatic syndromes" and "medically unexplained symptoms." Their reasoning is worth consideration, but I doubt the clinical utility of either rubric. The former is difficult to define, even by its proponents, but it draws on the idea that there is a spectrum of degrees to which normal people feel compelled to focus on unpleasant bodily sensations. At one end of the spectrum, the focusing becomes severe enough to warrant a diagnosis of "functional somatic syndrome." The other label, "medically unexplained symptoms," implies that the individual concerned would be better off if the symptoms were medically explicable. That promise thwarts the need to confront the psychosocial issues that compromise coping and serve to render the pain intolerable. However, the label "functional somatic syndromes" derives from important observations.

The people in the community who are burdened by persistent widespread pain, but have yet to avail themselves of a treatment act that labels them with fibromyalgia, suffer more than just chronic pervasive pain. Other everyday symptoms become momentous for them. Unlike the invincible person, people who are succumbing to the challenges of life and who use illness as a surrogate complaint seem to accumulate a host of unpleasant and unexpected bodily events. It appears that something must be dreadfully wrong. Some of these people quietly accept this sad state as their lot, but others vigorously cast about for an answer. The lay press and the Internet are at their service, as are many health-care professionals. Diagnostic terms such as Sjögren's, Raynaud's, lupus, Crohn's, fibromyalgia, chronic fatigue syndrome, TMJ syndrome, candida, EB virus, and many more are pressed into service. Many such sufferers seem convinced that their condition was sudden in onset, with a discrete cause, rather than being the slow erosion of their coping skills until some critical level of reserve became depleted. Many generate a causal hypothesis that takes on a life of its own and includes such attributions as "chemical imbalance," "virus," "stress," and "emotional confusion." According to a Canadian survey, most physiatrists, orthopaedists, and general practitioners are not convinced that fibromyalgia can be a consequence of or reactive to discrete events, including discrete traumatic events. Only some rheumatologists are comfortable with that hypothesis.

Functional somatic syndromes   Medical treatment acts are initiated on the basis of such histories. If it is with a primary care or specialty physician, the treatment will begin with a history of the present illness. In either case, a clinician predisposed to hearing certain complaints elicits the history. The primary care physician is prepared by previous experiences, the specialist by training. If you ask rheumatologists to examine the patients in a gastro-enterology clinic, for instance, they will diagnose fibromyalgia in the majority of patients previously diagnosed as suffering "irritable bowel syndrome" by the gastroenterologists. The gastroenterologists will return the favour if they examine the fibromyalgia patients in the rheumatology clinic and label them with irritable bowel syndrome. The symptoms of patients labelled with "chronic fatigue syndrome" overlap those of patients with fibromyalgia (the tender points as well), so as to render the distinction untenable. Hence, there is the argument that all these patients have a single "functional somatic syndrome" characterized by a spectrum of "medically unexplained symptoms." To me, another approach is to say that these people are predisposed to somatize when they are under stress, and this predisposition takes over their lives when they are overwhelmed by life's difficulties. Unfortunately, they are then rendered only more ill by the process of medicalization.

All of us somatize to some degree. I have written in the past that we all, at times, experience the "Syndrome of Out of Sorts." A "sort" was a device used by early printers to hold the letters of a single word or sentence together in typesetting. When we are "out of sorts," it seems as though the bits of our lives are coming unglued. On such occasions we feel "blue," or become aware of our bowels, or feel tired or stiff as if we have slept poorly. Sometime we know why, for challenges at home or at work are all too obvious. If we are concerned that our aggravating knee pain or backache or headache has returned, or is worse and harder to bear, we become even more out of sorts. Sometimes there is no known association – it just happens. Fortunately, it just passes, too. A bit of good news, a beautiful day, or an invigorating walk is often salving.

For some of us, feeling out of sorts is all too familiar. Some of us may be predisposed to somatizing because we carry an unusual sense of vulnerability. That may be the result of our upbringing. Some parenting styles create vulnerable children. These people are not "bad" parents, nor are their children disturbed. They are the kind of parents who, at the end of the day when they are tucking their children into bed, are inclined to the thought "Thank God Johnny made it today." They infect their child with a subtle, subliminal sense of impending doom. Such a pessimistic view of the world sometimes seems to run in families. Parents raise children to see the world as they do. The vulnerable child has been the subject of considerable academic interest in pediatrics for the past decade. This child grows up to be the vulnerable adult, for whom being out of sorts carries the weight of a self-fulfilling prophecy. Shaking off that sense of impending catastrophe is challenging, and the inability to do so has been labelled "catastrophizing." These are normal people, living life at one end of the spectrum of normal coping, and it is easy for them to trip up. The consequences of any such trip are easily modelled by the community in which they live or in the community they seek out. If they choose a medical recourse, medicalization and iatrogenicity may well be the result.

Several studies support this view. A World Health Organization survey found that 22 per cent of primary care patients around the world reported persistent pain. These patients were four times more likely to suffer anxiety or depression than patients without such pain, and even more likely to manifest unfavourable health perceptions than patients seeking care for other reasons. Another study done in Manchester, England, found that almost 5 per cent of the adult population reported chronic widespread pain. They were twice as likely as others to show psychological disturbance, limitations in function, and other somatic symptoms. Over time, the majority seemed to improve, though one-third showed no improvement despite their propensity to seek medical care.

If you have to prove you are ill, you can't get well Some circumstances in life predispose most, if not all, of us to somatize and catastrophize. Abusive relationships, job dissatisfaction, and job insecurity will do it, as will a worker's compensation claim for a chronically disabling regional musculoskeletal disorder (back pain, arm pain, or fibromyalgia in particular). Being a plaintiff in a personal injury lawsuit, a tort, will also do it. Whenever a person pursues an indemnity award for a disabling regional musculoskeletal disorder, from a back "injury" at work to "whiplash"-associated disorders, the claimant is expected to prove illness. Traditionally, the proof of illness has been subjugated to the proof of disease – to demonstrable tissue damage. If there is enough physical damage, and undisputed culpability, the symptoms are considered credible and an award follows efficiently. However, in the absence of sufficient "damage," a contest is joined which demands that the plaintiff or the claimant prove illness. For all the regional musculoskeletal disorders, most demonstrable "damage" is incidental and correlates little, if at all, with symptoms and function. Furthermore, by definition, regional musculoskeletal pain occurs in the course of activities that are customary and usually comfortable, so that culpability is seldom certain. These two features drive the claimant or plaintiff into a corner, beleaguered by adjusters and others who are demanding proof of specific damage and certain culpability rather than perceptions and beliefs. These individuals find themselves in a Kafkaesque vortex that causes them to somatize, magnify their symptoms, and acquire adverse illness behaviours.

Patients labelled with fibromyalgia are, by definition, spared any coincidental demonstrable specific damage. These people have to prove their illness in the absence of disease. The only way to do so depends on emotion and body language, levels of communication foreign to bureaucracies. The inevitable contest may be broached by the health insurer, who must approve treatment, or, more often, by an insurance carrier who needs to determine the magnitude of disability consequent to the fibromyalgia. Lawyers who serve the claimant recruit "experts," who find many tender points and espouse biomedical theories to explain the claimant's injury-related complaints. The insurer has a fiduciary responsibility to approve only effective treatments and to validate awards for disability. Lawyers for the insurer also recruit "experts," who find fewer tender points or who invoke alternative interpretations of the symptoms or the medical literature. The most predictable outcome is that the patient with the pervasive illness labelled fibromyalgia will get sicker and less capable of performing in society. That patient will focus on all the symptoms, recalling and often recording them at the instruction of legal counsel in a drive to document the magnitude of the illness. Symptom magnification is predictable. Since the veracity of the symptoms is at stake, any diminution in their intensity is made virtually impossible. Regression in intensity is tantamount to yielding to the insinuations that the symptoms were feigned in the first place. Illness escalates predictably. The other predictable outcome is that considerable wealth will be transferred from those who pay premiums to all those involved in this medicolegal process – with the exception, often, of the claimant, for whom pathos is the reward, and impoverishment the price to be paid.

Medicalization   The contest I've outlined plays out in a public arena. A more private contest awaits the person with persistent widespread pain who chooses to seek medical recourse. While less violent than the medicolegal contest, it is as likely to inflame the illness. This contest begins when the physician and the patient set out to define the biological "cause" of the persistent widespread pain as a prerequisite to treatment – a process that is bound to recruit the patient's undivided attention. The persistent widespread pain is then medicalized. The contest remains subliminal until the diagnostic process has proven fruitless, a time-consuming and anxiety-provoking exercise in testing, consulting, and running down false clues. The diminishing return of the diagnostic exercise is met with increasing tension in the patient-physician interaction. Any suggestions the doctor now offers about the value of psychological counselling are heard as accusations of the diagnosis "it's in your mind." The patient is placed in the position of proving to the physician that the pain is real – and proving the same to sceptics in the family, the social network, and the workplace. Such patients often recall and record symptoms in the course of the treatment act, just as they do in the course of a more public litigious contest. Their illness escalates. For these patients, caught in this vortex, the label fibromyalgia is much more than a diagnosis; it becomes a symbol of self-actualization. For me, or anyone else, to discuss its semiotics or to offer a sociocultural theory of pathogenesis is infuriating. That, too, is viewed as an assault on their veracity, an accusation that their symptoms are "in their mind."

One of the potentially dangerous acts physicians perform is to take a "history" from a patient. Physicians cannot avoid doing so, for the history provides the information needed to formulate a diagnosis, around which testing is structured. However, physicians tend to query in such a way that symptoms long ignored are revealed. Inevitably, the history medicalizes the symptoms so that they become the illness. To what end? Certainly there are occasions when crucial symptoms emerge from this process, ones that lead to a specific diagnosis, specific palliation, and even cure. In those instances, the medicalization of less-crucial symptoms is subsumed by the triumph of scientific medicine – that, at least, is the hope but probably the myth. Being a patient is a hazardous process. A person may sensibly consult a doctor for the treatment of acute bronchitis, only to learn during the course of healing that his PSA, or blood pressure, or blood glucose is elevated or that his customary nocturnal urination was noteworthy. In such circumstances, if the doctor is to avoid keeping patients unnecessarily as patients, rather than facilitating their return to personhood, she requires both skill and a sense of responsibility.

For patients with the complaint of persistent widespread pain, this taking of the history offers nothing but medicalization. Undoing that medicalization brings them full circle to the point made at the beginning of this chapter and the diagnosis "It's in your mind."

Mind-body duality   Why is this diagnosis so offensive? The answer relates to a social construction growing out of the sixteenth century. When William Harvey "discovered" the circulation of the blood, medicine and society could finally cast off the intellectual constraints of the Greek physician Galen. Vital humours were not amenable to testing, but science could contend with phenomena that were concrete, even measurable, such as Harvey's observation about blood. The workings of the body were open to study. The mind-body relationship was a different matter, however. Even the greatest philosopher-scientists and philosopher-physicians of the day could not cast off the abstraction of a "soul" or its cogitating handmaiden, a "mind." The "body" was composed of concrete, objective forms and structures that included the brain, but the mind and the soul were beyond ken. Yet, somehow, they must be connected to the physical reality of the body. René Descartes and his contemporaries went to lengths to infer the connection, usually relying on models of pain. Descartes was fascinated by the phenomenon of the "phantom limb," in which pain is perceived in an amputated limb. Sensations were the purview of the body, the nerves in particular, but pain was a higher function, a purview of the soul. It followed that pain, unaccompanied by correlative sensations in the body, should be considered like a phantom limb – a pain in the mind that is imaginary.

In the interests of brevity, I am not doing justice to this historiography. Cartesian thinking was far more involved. Others also had their versions of the mind-body duality: Sydenham conceived of an "internal man"; Blaise Pascal posited that "the ills of the body are nothing more than punishment [for the] ills of the soul"; Henry Cabinis, a French physician, conceived of a balance between pleasure and pain; while others argued variously from religious, metaphysical, psychological, or physiological perspectives. Over the centuries, the nature of pain caused, and still causes, considerable scientific and philosophical confusion. Philosophers have contended with the idea that pain might be not just evil but also useful. Western medicine has been taken to task more than once by a theological tradition of comforting to justify the inflicting of pain for some putative good, and it is still challenged on this basis.

Woven into these centuries of discourse and debate was the concept of hypochondria. In the early nineteenth century, Xavier Bichat, another French physician imbued with Cabinis's pain-pleasure duality, postulated that there were two "lives" – one inherent to the viscera, a vegetative life, and the other an interactive, conscious, and "animal" life. Hypochondria resulted when the normal painful, vegetative sensations, thought to be seated in the upper quadrants of the abdomen (the hypochondrium), moved across the threshold into conscious suffering. All this speculation might sound archaic, but modern psychology now terms this process "amplification" and recognizes Cabinis's "forces" as cognition, attention, context, and mood.

The label "hypochondriasis" is reserved for individuals with obsessive vigilance regarding bodily changes. These people can't notice a mole without thinking melanoma or note a palpitation without concluding heart disease. They establish a contract with medical providers, calling for the repeated reassurance of the diagnostic process. Medicalization is less an issue; no sense of invincibility is at risk. Modern psychiatry considers hypochondriasis at the extreme of a spectrum of "somatoform disorders" that afflict individuals who suffer from any physical symptom that defies medical explanation. If there are multiple symptoms, the term "somatization disorder" applies. These terms have superseded hysteria, conversion disorder, and a litany of discarded labels such as neurocirculatory asthenia, neuromyasthenia, and railway spine. However, all this labelling tends to belittle the symptoms and to stigmatize the patient. It is but a New Age form of "in your mind."

As important as the Cartesian mind-body duality paradigm was in pushing back the frontier of ignorance and metaphysical obfuscation in the seventeenth century, it is an impediment today. First, it is wrong. The mind is no longer an abstraction. Today we can probe it with single photon-emission computerized tomography (SPECT) scanning, forms of magnetic resonance (MR) imaging, and neurochemistry. We are starting to peel back the veils that shrouded the molecular basis of learning and emotion – and of nociception (the perception of pain beyond its sensation). The mind is no longer abstractly "that which thinks." Nociception involves receptors and transmitters and modulating electrophysiology. There is an underlying commonality to pain that makes it unspeakable, inexpressible in language, responsive to opiates, and reflexively aversive (so individuals automatically withdraw from situations causing it). The Cartesian mind-body duality no longer belongs in the clinic.

The Cartesian duality is perhaps being superseded by another duality. Pain does not involve only injury and physical disease. Pain recruits memory and cognition, and suffering recruits the psychosocial context of the afflicted individual. Nothing in life is as idiosyncratic as the experience of pain as suffering. If the pain-suffering duality could supplant the mind-body duality as the social construction, a Western patient could ask a Western physician "Is it in my mind?" without losing face.

8

Turning Aging into a Disease

Is greying a disease? I am not being facetious. Greying is a consequence of biological senescence, of growing old. The follicles that turn skin cells into hair have lost the capacity to introduce pigment. The loss of this biological function results in an obvious biological consequence. Is this consequence pathologic? If so, greying is a disease. If the consequence is not pathologic, greying is "normal."

Is greying an illness? For some, grey hair is a symptom, a biological event that is cause for concern and discomfit. For these people, greying is an illness, often an illness for which recourse is sought. The remedy is symptomatic, in that hair dyeing palliates the illness. The causal pathobiology of the follicle, the disease, is unchecked. Of course, for others, greying is not an illness, regardless of its underlying biology. These folks disregard the greying or find it pleasing, even distinguished. For them, it is one of many normal life transitions, as was puberty or pregnancy. They may find the underlying biology to be dramatic, but not pathologic. It's life.

To consider greying an illness is to "medicalize" it. As we discussed in the previous chapter, if the illness-disease paradigm is to be fulfilled, the underlying follicular biology must be pathologic. Greying is the illness one gets from diseased hair follicles. The syllogism calls for treatment of the disease to cure the greying. No doubt, if a wayward anti-hypertensive drug chanced to reinvigorate the production of pigment by hair follicles, as happened in the "cure" for balding, its manufacturer would be quick to petition the FDA for a licence. The drug would be eagerly marketed as the "cure" for greying. New subsections of august dermatology societies might form to discuss the breakthrough. Competing pharmaceutical firms would race to synthesize drugs with similar chemistry that would pass scrutiny by the FDA, at least in terms of convenience if not effectiveness. These firms would compete to underwrite educational programs for physicians and consumers alike. Advocacy organizations would seek to have the agents covered by Medicare.

Is this parody? Hardly.

OSTEOPENIA

For a generation or two, a small cadre of clinical investigators from several disciplines pursued the study of age-dependent changes in our bones. They enjoyed steady progress and a low profile – until recently. Today, the greying public lives in fear of shrinking away from "osteoporosis." Screening programs are recommended. Pharmaceutical firms are marketing aggressively to convince prescribers and consumers that they offer a product, by prescription or over the counter, that is the best choice. This enormous enterprise is bolstered by advocacy groups, professional societies, educational programs, and the like. Little is said about the choice to demur from screening, let alone to eschew chewing pills, ground oyster shells, or other potions. Almost no one is raising the issue of whether this entire enterprise is an egregious example of medicalization. This chapter will raise that issue.

The Age-Dependence of Mineralization

Bone is an extraordinary biological material. Its shape and resilience are properties of its protein matrix, most of which is collagen. Mineral salts, mainly calcium salts, incorporated into the matrix, give bone strength. Although the mineralized matrix is inert, bone is populated by cells specialized for its maintenance.

The composition of the resident cell population and the fine structure of the mineralized matrix are not uniform bone to bone. For example, the bones of the spine, the vertebrae, differ in important ways from both the femur and the skull. Each bone is a living organ. All bones are pre-programmed as to shape and architecture. Long bones and vertebrae respond to the habitual application of physical forces by compensatory changes in architecture. As is true of all organs in the human body, bones are continuously renewing themselves. The adult skeleton turns over every decade, though individual bones differ in this frequency. To achieve this progression, the bone cells must first demineralize the collagen and then degrade it while other cells are synchronized to replace the collagen in forms that facilitate remineralization with calcium salts. The tearing down is termed "resorption," and the rebuilding, "accretion." The entire process is called "remodelling."

Sometime after puberty, all our bones finish growing in length. However, they continue to "grow" in fine structure, gaining mineralized matrix well into our third or even fourth decade. This staging means that the remodelling results in a positive balance till we approach mid-life, when there is neither net gain nor loss. The degree of mineralization at mid-life is quite variable. On average, the plateau reached by women is less than that reached by men. Ancestral origin has a striking influence; bones of those with African roots are more mineralized than those with either Asian or European roots. A positive influence on the degree of mineralization can be achieved from moderate weight-bearing exercises, and a negative influence from thinness and tobacco abuse.

In our fifth decade, the balance turns negative. Slowly we come to have less mineral per unit matrix and, therefore, less well-mineralized bone. In men, this negative balance is a gentle slope that continues until death. In women, the negative balance accelerates with menopause. On the whole, though, there is considerable variability in the rate of demineralization between people and within the skeleton. The bones whose articulating ends (joints) have osteoarthritis are, relatively, spared demineralization. So are the bones of individuals who have more fatty tissue, who have avoided cigarette smoking, and who exercise regularly. But the sparing is relative; demineralization is "normal."

Bone that is less well mineralized is more fragile. Very few well people demineralize to the degree that important fractures are unavoidable, however – and our discussion in this book is aimed at well people. The drugs and diseases that drive demineralization are beyond our scope. However, some people demineralize sufficiently to incur a significant risk of fracture. The jargon terms this status as "osteopenia," meaning scant bone. If someone with osteopenia suffers a fracture without an extraordinary physical exposure, the fracture is termed a "pathological fracture," and the underlying disease is termed osteoporosis, denoting a pathological degree of osteopenia. Extrapolating from our discussion of the plateaus of mineralization, the people most at risk are found among thin women of European or Asian ancestry, but no one is spared some degree of risk.

Pathological Fractures

Osteopenia is never an illness. People never know that their bones are demineralizing. The issue is the disease – pathological fractures. Reasonably, people might want to know if their osteopenia is severe enough to put them at sufficiently high risk of a pathological fracture to justify trying to restore mineralization. However, this request assumes that an intervention exists which has proved to be effective and has a favourable benefit/risk ratio. If the intervention were effective with trivial risk, perhaps it would be sensible for everyone to partake of its beneficence regardless of the degree of osteopenia. Such was the basis for the public health policy of fluoridation of drinking water to prevent dental caries. However, if the intervention is of uncertain beneficence, or the benefit/risk ratio is indeterminate or marginal, should one intervene simply because osteopenia imparts risk? As it stands, the interventions for osteopenia are of uncertain benefit across the board. For some, the benefit/risk ratio is not known but likely unfavourable, while for others the interventions approach the trivial. Before we examine these interventions, we should first understand more about the disease of osteoporosis and its principle manifestation – pathological fractures.

Three regions of our skeleton carry this risk: the spine, the proximal femur (hip), and the distal forearm (near the wrist). Pathologic fractures from primary osteoporosis elsewhere are too rare to factor into the decision to screen and intervene for osteopenia.

Pathological Fractures of the Spine   The scientific, clinical, and lay literatures relating to osteoporotic pathological fractures of the spine treat the topic as if there were no other spine disorders affecting the elderly. They give the impression that banishing osteopenia would free the elderly of axial morbidity. Nothing could be further from the truth. All elderly people have degenerative diseases of the spine. They all cope with backache frequently. Many surveys suggest that persistent backache affects up to 50 per cent of women over the age of sixty-five. Osteoporotic pathological fractures are a minor factor in all this morbidity.

Part of the degenerative process leads to the loss of discs, the soft tissue structures separating the vertebrae. Few over the age of sixty-five have not suffered this change at more than one spinal level, though, as we discussed in chapter 6, the presence of such degenerative changes correlates very poorly with symptoms. However, these changes always exact a penalty on the height of the individual. Inches are lost as we age because of loss of the disc spacing.

That's the area where osteoporotic compression fractures play out. Nearly all compression fractures occur in the thoracic portion of the spine, particularly affecting the vertebrae between the shoulder blades. The vertebrae are normally cylinders. If they are osteopenic, the endplates of the bony cylinder can collapse, creating "codfish" vertebrae, so-called because they acquire the shape of fish vertebrae. This type of fracture has little consequence in terms of posture. However, if the anterior wall (the wall facing forward) collapses, the cylinder assumes a wedge shape, creating a forward-leaning curve to the thoracic spine – a kyphosis, or "dowager's hump." The result is additional loss in stature and some degree of deformity.

Both degenerative changes and backache are ubiquitous in the elderly, but compression fractures are rare. If you identify a thousand women in their seventies who have no compression fractures on spine x-rays and follow them for a year, approximately fifteen will develop a compression fracture. Women with one compression fracture are several times more likely to have a new compression fracture in the following year.

Is this all there is to osteoporosis, a condition analogous to greying? Because of degenerative changes, all of us lose stature, all of us lose flexibility, and all of us tend towards kyphosis. Some people age in this fashion more than others, just as some assume a distinctive posture. Are these changes simply concomitants of aging, or is there more to them? Is there an illness that results from these compression fractures?

Although this anatomical change is a "fracture," most patients can recall no distinctive episode of pain that led to it, and most are incidental findings on chest x-rays. Occasionally a patient presents with acute severe back pain between the shoulder blades, with a coincident compression fracture. The association is tenable, since this presentation is unusual except in the elderly. Most episodes of acute back pain are in the low back. This syndrome of acute compression fracture is a miserable experience, particularly because it may be prolonged and difficult to palliate. Fortunately, it tends to be self-limited; it gets better on its own, though there is a tendency for a recurrence or two. However, this acute compression fracture syndrome is an exceptional presentation for a disease that is not particularly prevalent in the first place. Population studies show very little association between an increase in back symptoms and an increase in the prevalence or incidence of compression fractures. They show but a suggestion of such a link, and that may reflect the occasional case of the acute syndrome. Even if we did manage to prevent spinal compression fractures, then, it would have only a limited impact on the burden of spinal pain or pathoanatomy in the aging population.

Hip Fractures   Hip fracture is serious. Pathologic hip fractures are not the same as compression fractures, though both can occur in the course of normal activities. Spinal compression fractures are generally asymptomatic, meaning the symptoms they engender are perceived as yet another of the intermittent and remittent axial pains that are a common experience in the elderly. Pathologic hip fractures, in contrast, are never subsumed under the labels of the usual musculoskeletal disorders. They are painful and, because they halt weight bearing, they affect mobility. Coping is not an option unless the patient takes to bed for the rest of his life. It would seem, then, that hip fractures should be a compelling argument for the treatment of osteopenia, but they are not – and for good reason.

Hip fractures are easy to fix. There are surgical options, the commonest of which, pinning, is straightforward and requires little post-operative rehabilitation. One of the paradoxes of the circumstance of osteoporotic hip fractures is that the "cure" is both easy and Pyrrhic. Most osteoporotic pathologic hip fractures are the fate of the elderly, but only some of the elderly. If you follow a thousand Dutch women in their eighth decade for a year, for example, five will suffer a hip fracture. If you follow a subset of Dutch women of that same age who are particularly osteopenic, the likelihood of hip fracture doubles or triples. It is not simply a matter of chance. The women who suffer the fractures are frailer and more likely to fall. Frail women and men who have osteoporotic hip fractures have markedly decreased longevity and functionality, despite the fact that their fractures are expeditiously and safely managed. Fall-induced injuries are increasing in older adults at a rate that cannot be explained by demographic changes. The increase may result from the many medications they consume with side effects that compromise mobility, stability, and alertness. The frail elderly should be individually assessed for behavioural interventions such as exercise programs and for modifications of environmental hazards that can help to reduce falls. Vanity aside, the most effective intervention to prevent osteoporotic hip fractures is for the frail elderly to wear a padded corset. No other intervention has proven as effective in decreasing the likelihood and severity of falling.

Colles Fractures   Osteoporotic fractures of the distal forearm, or wrist, are not really "pathological" because they are always a consequence of trauma. The typical story is that breaking a fall with the extended wrist breaks the distal forearm. As was the case for osteoporotic hip fractures, the first principle of treatment is to avoid falls. For the elderly, particularly the frail elderly, that solution often requires more than advice. It is important that the living area be unencumbered by objects and surfaces likely to trip the dweller up. Assistive devices might be necessary to stabilize gait and transfers: canes, walkers, elevated seats, and the like. Balance and stability of the elderly can also be improved with training and practice. It is all part of achieving the "ripe old age" we will discuss in the epilogue.

To return to the "greying hair" analogy, pathologic fractures are a disease that is likely to increase with the degree of osteopenia. However, in the case of spinal compression fractures, the illness that can be ascribed to this disease is quite variable. Most often there is none. Sometimes the illness is considerable, an acute compression fracture syndrome, but transient. Sometimes there is an alteration in posture beyond the expected level in the peer group and causing some deformity. For spinal compression fractures, the benefit/risk ratio to proactively treat osteopenia must be convincingly favourable. Nearly all well people who are fortunate to live long enough to contend with the spectre of spinal compression fractures will not have to contend with the reality.

For osteoporotic hip and wrist fractures, more leniency in the risk/benefit ratio is acceptable, but not much. If attention is given to reducing the risk of falling, there is little more to be gained. To gain that little more, risk should not be tolerated.

However, families and managers of residential facilities for the elderly need to be aware that complex interventions that are based on individual health assessments can reduce falls. These should include behavioural interventions and modifications of environmental hazards.

Meddling with Osteopenia

Given these benefit/risk considerations, let's examine the marketed menu of remedies in order of acceptability.

Dietary Supplements Calcium and vitamin D supplements top this list. These preparations are offered over the counter, are sold aggressively in stores and in the media, and form part of the enormous North American vitamin scam. The average person eating an average diet in any industrialized country has no need for vitamin or mineral supplements. For most well people, there is no discernible benefit, but there is little risk either. I have no argument with people who seek out and avail themselves of unproved remedies, or even those proven to be worthless, as long as the putative remedies are harmless and I don't have to share the expense via my health insurance premiums or tax dollars. Several vitamins, notably vitamins D and A, are anything but harmless, however, if they are taken in excess.

The average person receives no benefit from calcium and vitamin D supplements because our endocrine system monitors the blood level of calcium and maintains it at exactly our personal set point. Our calcium absorption is tightly controlled to that end. The mechanism is elegant. If the blood calcium level trends down, vitamin D is converted to an active metabolite, which makes the intestinal absorption of calcium more efficient, and vice versa. No matter how much calcium you ingest, the fraction absorbed will be controlled to reflect the blood calcium level. The same holds for the activation of most forms of vitamin D, including the form produced by sunlight exposure to our skin. It is estimated that about an hour in the mid-day sun will generate our daily requirement. Unlike calcium, it is possible to overdose with all the available vitamin D preparations.

There may be subsets of normal, well people in advanced countries who are at risk for a dietary insufficiency of calcium or vitamin D. In theory at least, people who avoid dairy products and have a lower calcium intake and less vitamin D supplementation should be at risk for osteopenia. However, such a subset is difficult to tease out of the general population. Perhaps these individuals have adequate calcium intake from other sources or are predisposed to sun exposure. The data to support a public health recommendation about dairy food consumption are quite inconsistent, and any such recommendation is controversial. However, there is one subset of well people for whom a diet deficient in calcium or vitamin D is a risk for osteopenia. That subset is the elderly, particularly the institutionalized elderly and, most particularly, institutionalized or homebound elderly women. Frail individuals most likely to suffer osteoporotic hip fractures are likely to be malnourished generally, including in calcium and vitamin D. Clearly, nutrition, environmental modifications, and behavioural interventions all deserve attention in designing a milieu that promotes bone health in the elderly.

Hormone Replacement Therapy   HRT is next in our hierarchy of acceptability for meddling with osteopenia – in spite of the recent brouhaha over its use. Menopause is a biological passage. For a generation of women, it has been followed by a rite of passage – the decision to continue menstruating in the absence of ovulation. This decision is never prejudiced by some need to continue menstruating. Rather, HRT was foisted on the post-menopausal woman under the widely advertised banner of prolonging youthfulness. The medicalization of menopause was a goldmine both for gynecologists and for the pharmaceutical firms that manufacture and market estrogen-containing compounds. Undoubtedly, HRT can have beneficial effects on vaginal dryness and perimenopausal symptoms, which can occasionally be devastating. However, the former responds to topical estrogen, and the latter to brief exposure to low-dose estrogen. Nonetheless, the benefits of long-term HRT became a social construction that continues to sway as many as 40 per cent of post-menopausal women. They were swayed initially by the promise of an improved quality of life, and then by the promise of a lessened risk of osteoporosis and its disabling consequences. The latter follows from the observation in 1941 by Fuller Albright, a pioneer of modern endocrinology, that menopause was associated with spinal osteoporosis – for which he recommended estrogen therapy. The promise of HRT did not stop there. After all, there are many diseases that spare pre-menopausal women and afflict post-menopausal women, and HRT, it was thought, might prove to be the salve. Heart disease was suggested, to name one.

For nearly thirty years, epidemiology has picked away at the associations between HRT and clinical outcomes. The quality-of-life myth has proven unsupportable except for perimenopausal symptoms. One study suggests that HRT increases the risk of back pain. Although HRT had been shown to decrease the rate of bone mineral loss, no compelling effect on the fracture rate has been demonstrated. Multiple trials examining cardiovascular outcomes have yielded inconsistent results, perhaps an increased risk that is transient with the institution of HRT. Some increased risk of thrombophlebitis and pulmonary embolism seemed to emerge, along with an increased risk of breast and uterine cancer with prolonged exposure to HRT. However, the many studies on all these associations had inconsistencies and small effects.

Despite little or no evidence in its favour, HRT consumption continued at much the same level. Then the results were published of the randomized controlled trial of the risks and benefits of estrogen plus progestin (the combination HRT most commonly prescribed) from the Women's Health Initiative. Between 1993 and 1998 this initiative recruited some 162,000 post-menopausal women into a set of clinical trials sponsored and monitored by the National Institutes of Health and conducted at forty centres across the United States. The HRT component involved 16,000 of these women, selected because they had not had their uteruses surgically removed. They were randomly assigned to take HRT or not. After 5.2 years, the investigators charged to monitor the trial outcomes considered the results to be so dramatic, if not horrifying, that they felt duty bound to stop the trial early. The health risks exceeded the health benefits (see table 8.1). In the summer of 2002 the world

Table 8.1
Women's Health Initiative HRT Randomized Controlled Trial

Health Outcome	Relative Risk	Absolute Risk (events per 10,000 people per year)
Heart disease	29% increase	7 more
Invasive breast cancer	26% increase	8 more
Stroke	41% increase	8 more
Pulmonary embolism	113% increase	8 more
Hip fracture	34% decrease	5 less
Colorectal cancer	37% decrease	6 less

press heralded this result. The powerful HRT social construction has been tottering ever since.

Much of the media talk was of the relative risks. It sounds awful that HRT causes a 41 per cent increased risk of stroke, but in terms of absolute risk it means that 8 of 10,000 women will suffer a stroke because they took HRT for a year. That is a gamble many might take if they believed their youthfulness and vitality were at stake. Some might argue that the tradeoff with hip fractures and colorectal cancer makes the hazards more tolerable. After all, there were no extra deaths ascribable to HRT; most women sailed through their cardiac event, recovered from their stroke, or were "cured" of their breast cancer – if we believe the predictions set out in the relevant chapters in Part One of this book. There's also the question we discussed earlier of the reliability and validity of small differences detected in huge trials. In short, the benefit/risk assessment of HRT remains imponderable. But why should anyone prescribe such an agent? Even the US Preventive Services Task Force, which held up releasing its updated recommendations until they could be revised in light of these results, can find no justification for the routine use of HRT. Further analyses of the results of the Women's Health Initiative have reinforced the finding that there is a slight (0.5%) increase in the absolute risk for stroke, and a smaller increase in the risk for cognitive impairment.

Perhaps the death knell for treating post-menopausal women with HRT will come less from the litany of tiny hazards than from the analysis of the quality of life of the women who participated in the Women's Health Initiative. In this placebo-controlled

randomized trial, the women on HRT and the women on placebo were indistinguishable in terms of general health, vitality,
mental health, depressive symptoms, or sexual satisfaction. So
much for the HRT social construction!

At the same time that the post-menopausal population taking
HRT are being pummelled by these statistically significant,
though tiny, hazards, they are being aggressively marketed as to
putatively less-concerning pharmaceutical alternatives for meddling with osteopenia. A selective estrogen-receptor modulator
(SERM) is already available in the pharmacy. Estrogen binds with
two forms of receptors to initiate its biological effects, so pharmaceutical firms have been synthesizing molecules that compete
with estrogen for these receptors. Two kinds are available. One,
tamoxifen, effectively blocks the receptor. Tamoxifen is an agent
used to treat breast cancer, and it has been studied in large trials
on the prevention of breast cancer (which discerned marginal
and balancing risks and benefits). One concern in these trials
was that blocking the estrogen receptor would predispose the
women to osteopenia, if not osteoporosis, but, surprisingly, that
concern did not materialize. Another compound, raloxifene
(marketed as Evista), is structurally similar to tamoxifen and also
binds estrogen receptors. However, raloxifene preferentially targets receptors in the cells in bone and, rather than blocking,
effectively activates those receptors.

The hope is that a SERM of this type might prevent osteopenia
by estrogen effects on bone without stimulating the uterine
endometrium. Thus, both menstruation and any increased risk
of uterine cancer might be avoided. The manufacturer underwrote a multicentre randomized controlled trial, first recruiting
lead investigators (many of whom avowed financial arrangements within the pharmaceutical industry) and then recruiting
over 7,000 women. After three years, the women on raloxifene
had less osteopenia. Those women who had no vertebral fractures at the beginning of the trial had no meaningful reduction
in new vertebral compression fractures after three years (there
was a significant difference but it was tiny). However, for women
who had fractures at inception, the reduction was over 5 per

cent. There was no reduction in hip fractures. There was a tradeoff in leg cramps, hot flashes, edema, and flu-like symptoms, but none in terms of cardiovascular events. Much ado about nothing? The FDA didn't think so. However, I never prescribe a new compound unless the benefit/risk ratio is compelling. I am unwilling to expose my patients to uncertainties regarding long-term consequences unless there is a compelling tradeoff with short-term benefits. In the discussion above, is the reduction in the incidence of spinal compression fractures a compelling benefit?

Those who argue for treating osteopenia with a SERM reserve therapy for people at higher risk for spinal compression fractures. This subset can be identified because either they already have a spinal compression fracture or they have a greater degree of osteopenia. This argument has been better developed for another class of agents, the bisphosphonates.

Pipe Cleaners   In the 1960s, chemical engineers at Proctor & Gamble solved a problem that had long plagued the manufacture of soap. The effluent from the process of saponification was rich in calcium salts, which formed concretions in the plumbing. The engineers came across a class of small calcium-binding molecules, the bisphosphonates, which could keep the pipes clear.

There is a rare hereditary disorder, myositis ossificans, which causes muscle to turn to bone. In the 1960s, before legal and FDA constraints were fully in place, a well-read clinician treated a patient devastated by this disease with a bisphosphonate. He published a promising anecdote. Unfortunately for that patient and others with this rare disease, the anecdote does not reproduce. However, the fact that this class of agent was not intrinsically toxic opened the door to inventive chemistry and clinical investigation. The pharmaceutical division of Proctor & Gamble has been a leader in this area.

It was soon discovered that bisphosphonates had totally different effects on human biology than on industrial plumbing. They did not bind calcium. However, they did have interesting and varied effects on the resident populations of cells in bone. Etidronate was one of the earliest bisphosphonates to make its way in clinical medicine when it was used in the treatment of Paget's disease of bone, a condition in which the unbridled resorption of bone outstrips the formation of proper new bone so that remodelling is disorganized. Etidronate slows the resorption and improves remodelling. It also slows resorption of normal bone, thereby thwarting post-menopausal osteopenia. However, it is not easy to use for that purpose because, at higher doses, it also interferes with the renewal process, leading to osteopenic bone by another mechanism. In practice today, the agent is prescribed for two weeks out of every two months for two years. Trials suggest that this regimen is about as effective as the SERM we just discussed; the incidence of vertebral fractures is reduced by about 5 per cent over two years of treatment. That's an absolute reduction of 5 per cent. There is no demonstrable effect on the incidence of hip or other non-vertebral fractures. However, more intense or more prolonged dosing causes, rather than thwarts, osteopenia. You have to be wary of all bisphosphonates as double-edged swords. One agent, for example, was withdrawn from the market because it caused leukemia as a side effect.

The experience with etidronate was favourable enough for Proctor & Gamble and its competitors to pursue new bisphosphonates for the prevention of osteopenia. Already, several are on the market and many more are in development. Two bisphosphonates introduced in the late 1990s now compete to dominate the market. The competition plays out in advertising campaigns aimed at professionals and at consumers. All these marketing dollars are highly visible in "continuing education" programs and in sponsorship of professional meetings. If anything is shoring up the osteoporosis social construction, it is this effort, coupled with industry-sponsored research protocols that are far more effective in inserting these agents into medical practice styles than in pushing back the frontier of medical ignorance. Women are increasingly aware of and fret about the fate of their skeletons. Machines designed to measure their degree of osteopenia (vide infra) abound. And many women who feel and are well are consuming these expensive bisphosphonates

Table 8.2
Number of Fractures at Different Sites over Three Years in the VERT Trial

Treatment	Wrist	Hip	Arm	Leg	Clavicle
Risedronate	14	12	4	4	3
Placebo	22	15	10	8	0

because their bone mineral density (BMD) is said to offer them no better choice.

The two agents are alendronate (marketed by Merck as Fosamax) and risedronate (marketed by Procter & Gamble as Actonel). Both experienced difficulty in getting approval at the FDA. The randomized placebo-controlled trials that convinced the FDA to license these two agents were similar in design: multi-centre, inception cohorts of thousands of post-menopausal women, and follow-up for several years while monitoring BMD and the incidence of fractures. Both agents have a measurable therapeutic effect on BMD. For women with previous vertebral fractures, or a relatively low BMD, both agents decrease the incidence of vertebral fractures to the same degree – an absolute reduction in incidence of about 5 per cent over at least three years of observation. Not surprisingly, the publications and the marketing emphasize the *relative* reductions, which get up to 40 per cent because the incidence in the placebo groups is around 10 per cent. These fractures are defined as a 15 per cent decrease in the height of a vertebra for risedronate, and 20 per cent for alendronate – not as a decrease in the incidence of acute pain or the likelihood of an important alteration in posture. Risedronate is reasonably safe and well tolerated in the short run. Alendronate ran into problems with irritation of the esophagus. Merck has partially circumvented this toxicity by altering the dosing schedule from daily to weekly, but that change was made after licensing by the FDA. Both agents are also marketed as effective in the prevention of non-vertebral fractures, but that claim begs circumspection. Table 8.2 sets out the data from the pivotal 1999 risedronate trial, the "VERT" trial.

This study randomized 1,600 post-menopausal women for three years. The risk of non-vertebral fracture is small in the placebo group, an incidence of 3 per cent for wrist fractures and 2 per cent for hip fractures. It is difficult to measure a meaningful reduction with such a low incidence. The claim is for an overall reduction in non-vertebral fractures: thirty-seven incurred by women taking risedronate, and fifty-five by those on placebo. There is no statistical difference in hip fractures. Osteoporotic fractures of the arm and leg are far less frequent than hip fractures in the population, so this placebo population is not representative. In that regard, these women were unlucky. I have combed the published trial data that tests the assertion that treatment with alendronate or risedronate for several years reduces the hip fracture rate, even in women with moderately severe osteopenia, and it is not impressive. As for the women with clinically severe osteopenia, who already have asymptomatic vertebral compression fractures or have suffered symptomatic spinal or other osteoporotic fractures, the argument to treat them with HRT or a bisphosphonate is more compelling. However, even in this circumstance, the clinical context is our master. In the frail elderly, what is to be gained?

Measuring BMD   I have postponed discussing the measurement of BMD in order to first inform the reader about its tenuous rationale. Measuring BMD has become another rite of passage for women of all ages. Even young, fair-skinned, menstruating, recreational athletes are now made to worry about osteopenia. Screening is advertised, promoted, urged, and advised in print, voice, and broadcast media, in health clubs and health magazines, and in many a professional office. Determining BMD is big business and largely bogus. No one should be screened for any disease, ever, unless the test is accurate, the result has meaningful predictive value, and there is something meaningful to be done if the test is positive. BMD measurement fails on all accounts.

Most "store front" BMD measurements are performed by DEXA scanning – dual energy x-ray absorptiometry. This technique is both difficult to standardize and subject to many technical errors. There are other kinds of measurements on the market, and many discussions of which anatomical site is most predictive.

Most of the data we have discussed were based on DEXA scans at the hip and spine. You can do better using variations on computerized tomography (CT), but that assumes you can justify devoting such expensive hardware to this exercise.

Any measured value short of the extremes of osteopenia has very little predictive value in people under the age of sixty. No well woman under that age should even consider this test. The US Preventive Services Task Force avoided this population, unwilling to recommend for or against, in its 2002 recommendations, as did the authors of an influential review of the same year in the *Journal of the American Medical Association,* authors who have been leading investigators on the alendronate trials and so have a relationship with Merck. These authors suggest that a tradeoff in "changes in behaviors that might decrease fracture risk" might justify rendering a young woman "unnecessarily anxious about a low result." But should these women exercise more to increase bone density, or exercise less to gain in body mass index (BMI), since that, too, correlates with increased BMD? Both the task force and the alendronate investigators favour screening after the age of sixty-five and, for women with "risk factors" such as a low BMI in white women, between the ages of sixty and sixty-five. Anyone with a low BMD should be treated. This recommendation is echoed by all kinds of professional organizations, from the National Osteoporosis Foundation to the professional bodies for orthopaedics, endocrinology, geriatrics, and more. It departs from the recommendation against such universal screening of a consensus conference sponsored by the National Institutes of Health and published in 2000.

Am I wrong in doubting the advice of these professional bodies that universal screening with BMD meets the three criteria above? While we all agree with those criteria, the differences hinge on the distinction between clinically significant and statistically significant. The pro-measurement experts base their recommendations on the latter; I base mine on the former. Universal screening at the age of sixty-five cannot be defended because its predictive value is marginal. Indeed, based on the trivial, or arguable, magnitude of benefit that has been demonstrated in the

wealth of therapeutic trials, even if it were possible to predict risk
accurately, the clinical benefit would be tenuous. I am not alone
in my scepticism. The US Agency for Healthcare Research and
Quality convened a panel to write guidelines, which were published in 2001 and justified my scepticism. The charge to this
government agency was to perform analytic literature reviews in
the name of evidence-based medicine. It is now defunct, subsumed into a larger agency with a different agenda. However, its
deliberations are precious.

OSTEOPENIA: A SOCIAL CONSTRUCTION

Research articles on this topic usually state that osteoporosis is
important because it is common, causes substantial morbidity,
and costs over several billion dollars per year. Yet very few authors
question whether this construction is medicalization of aging
and wonder whether this price tag is part of the unconscionable
American way of dying (as we will discuss in the epilogue). Perhaps many Americans, particularly the more advantaged American women, have bought into this construct. Furthermore, in
accepting that screening and treatment make sense, they have
done more than buy into an idea. The construction has become
a commonly and tightly held tenet – a social construction.

Many wait with bated breath for the next breakthrough. With
the announcement that zoledronic acid, a bisphosphonate,
could be given intravenously once a year for the prevention of
osteopenia, the press and Novartis stockholders took notice.
When Eli Lilly's new pharmaceutical, a parathyroid hormone
fragment, was shown to prevent osteopenia and even diminish
the incidence of osteoporotic fractures, medicine and Wall Street
took notice. It seems sensible that all this effort be expended,
that all white women and maybe others, at the age of sixty-five
and maybe younger, rejoice at the progress of science. Social
constructions are not "bad." Daily life abounds in them, in belief
systems that have yet to be refuted. For many such social constructions, the idea that they are refutable seems absurd. Each
culture, each era, has operational social constructions and it

always will. We have already seen several examples that relate to health in this book. Other social constructions relate to behaviours, "race," income distribution, and much more, and any among them seem to have had a finite life expectancy. History marks some that passed quietly, and others that left scars. Some have a life of their own, and others are resilient in spite of the assault of science. The concept of race is an example, surviving for over a century in spite of its tragic history and the recent scientific pummelling.

Osteopenia is an example of a New Age social construction, propelled to its status in a decade by aggressive marketing and vested interests. It has been tested, and is being tested, and has proven marginal, if not untenable. It has also proven resilient. Much is vested in that staying power by all the providers. It may even become a "meme" (rhymes with "gene") – a recent term to describe an *idée fixe* that is infectious. The proponents of the concept of a "meme" even postulate some biological reality, some infectious unit of knowledge or of memory. I'll settle for a more psychological conceptualization. Memes insert themselves into the very being of the infected, so fibromyalgia, for example, is a meme for the susceptible. It is very difficult to alter a social construction, but even more difficult to ablate a meme. Has osteopenia, along with other fashionable illnesses, become a meme?

9

Health Hazards in the Hateful Job

Some of the hazards to our well-being lurk in the course of living. They are aspects of our interactive worlds, our ecosystems, that can perturb our biology and control our fate. Two have emerged that are particularly powerful and that threaten our longevity far more than such recognized causes as hypertension, obesity, or adult onset diabetes. Both of these life-course hazards relate to impediments to the pursuit of gainful employment.

A lifetime tottering on the edge of poverty is a lifetime likely to be mean, often discouraging, sometimes desperate – and also short. What is it about a compromised socioeconomic status (SES) that is so malevolent? Multiple psychosocial factors have emerged from the studies of relative poverty. Some of these factors operate from conception, but the majority derive from the loss of self-respect and the resentment, if not hostility, that results from the sense of abject vulnerability associated with and imposed by poverty. A few are associated with nutrition and life-stage maturation. Much remains unknown, but it is clear that the array of psychosocial challenges to be faced day after day in poverty, and that prove insurmountable, levy a heavier toll on health and longevity than any other factor in the "advanced" world. Poverty in nations that are not resource-challenged is a reproach to both their political systems and their public health agendas.

Employment itself is no generic solution to the malevolence of poverty. Some facets of life in modern workforces rival the psychosocial aspects of poverty in extracting a toll on healthfulness and longevity. A consistent story is starting to emerge, with major implications for the health of the public.

Do you like your job? Are you valued at work? These two questions deserve a prominent place in the body politic and in whatever caring community life affords us. They should anchor a major public health initiative. Negative answers to these questions are associated with clinical morbidity and affect longevity even for those who could, if they wished, change their jobs. For growing numbers of workers, however, job mobility is not an option or it can lead only to less-acceptable alternatives. Particularly for the aging workforce, who began their career assuming job security, the insecurity of the current labour market comes as a surprise.

For all of us, life presents challenges to coping. In addition to challenges in relationships and with employment, we experience variations in mood, intermittent musculoskeletal discomfort, occasional headaches, episodic respiratory symptoms, and remittent physical distress. To be well, to feel invincible, is to have the personal wherewithal to cope with both the physical and the psychosocial challenges. When overwhelmed, we transform our distress into narratives that are culturally defined and constrained. Our Western culture predisposes us to frame any loss of a sense of well-being or other forms of psychosocial distress into idioms of physical, rather than psychosocial, distress. As we have seen, the possibility that psychosocial confounders exacerbate any aspect of our infirmity is anathema, tantamount to the condemnation "It's in your head!" So we leap to the conclusion that the reason we can't cope relates to the intensity of the physical distress. Sometimes we're correct, but more often it's the psychosocial challenges, not the physical, that are primary. In the workforce, misconceptions about the physical cause of regional musculoskeletal disorders have misled the occupational health and safety agenda for over sixty years.

Regional musculoskeletal disorders account for the preponderance of long-term disability in the workforce. Regional backache is now rivalled by regional arm pain as the scourge of the Western workforce. Since motion can exacerbate these symptoms, the

contemporary industrialized world is quick to ascribe any associated work incapacity to the physical content of tasks at work. It
was not always so. Understanding how it came to be, and what it
represents, is essential to understanding why disabling regional
musculoskeletal disorders are a window into the quality of life in
the workforce and, simultaneously, the hazards to healthfulness
and longevity that appear when that quality is compromised.

THE ERGONOMIC SOCIAL CONSTRUCTION

"Why me?" This plaint pertains to all illness. In less-enlightened,
more complicated times long past, the sufferer was likely to light
on such answers as fate or, perhaps, retribution for ill-advised
behaviour. The Elizabethan explanation for backache included
requital for dissipation, if Shakespeare's *Measure for Measure* bears
witness. Attribution has superseded retribution as a comfortable
explanation only in the past century. Before then, tasks had to
be "back breaking" before it seemed reasonable to ascribe backache to them. It is still more customary to blame "a pain in the
neck" on the behaviour of another person than on one's own
activities. To "shoulder a burden" remains less a condemnation
than a designation of fortitude.

Before attribution could supersede retribution as the accepted
cause for backache, new social constructions had to come into
place. First came the invention of "railway spine" in the nineteenth century and its promulgation as a Victorian medicalization by John Eric Erichsen, a professor of surgery in University
College, London. The railroad was one of the engines of industrialization. Building railroads was dangerous work, and too
often maiming or lethal work. Even riding the rails was dangerous; collisions and derailments were so commonplace that
Queen Victoria insisted that her private train travel very slowly.
However, consternation about the carnage on the early railway
did not surface till the turn of the century. What first captured
the mass psyche was the illness that befell passengers who had
been spared violent events – a pervasive debilitating illness
notable for axial myalgias and fatigue. Erichsen explained it as

"concussion of the spine from slight injury." Victorian England reeled from the condemnation and subsequent litigation of this social construction. Towards the end of his life, however, Erichsen withdrew his support from this theory, and railway spine disappeared. It left as its legacy the common belief that people can be "injured" during the course of customary activities and without unusual trauma. Backache was firmly established as a medical problem.

The demise of railway spine coincided with the birth of workers' compensation indemnity schemes. This legislation provides redress for the injuries and fatalities resulting from industrialization, including the building and maintenance of railroads. Prussian social legislation created the template that exists throughout the industrial world to this day. It entitles workers to medical care and wage replacement if they suffer accidental injuries that arise out of, and in the course of, employment. In the absence of a violent precipitant, backache was not scheduled as a compensable "injury" for the early decades of the twentieth century. That changed in 1934, when W.J. Mixter and J.S. Barr had the temerity to label extrusion of nucleus pulposus (the soft central part of the intervertebral disc) a "rupture of the intervertebral disc" – a semiotic that Barr was to recant late in his career. The implication of "rupture" was so violent that the word alone classified any sufferer as injured. In that way a regional backache that interfered with work, particularly when ascribed to a ruptured disc or if lamina had been surgically violated, became a compensable back "injury." In similar fashion, society has accepted that the label "rupture" can pertain to an inguinal hernia. To this day, the United States leads the "advanced" world in the likelihood of doing surgical violence to the lumbosacral spines of workers with compensable regional back "injuries." The incidence varies from region to region, with some communities contriving surgical indications ten times more frequently than others.

Rutherford Johnstone described the social construction of the "industrial back" nicely in 1941 in his book *Occupational Diseases*: "In complete disregard of the multiple causes of backache," he wrote, "the tendency in industrial medicine is to 'mass-group' all these cases under the diagnosis of back sprain. This error seems to be predicated upon the 'locale' of the onset of pain. If it ensues while a man is cutting his own lawn, the term 'lumbago' is invariable applied and the condition attributed to causes within the man. But pain arising while stooping, bending, or lifting at the plant is called 'back sprain' and considered the result of motion while working for someone else. The situation assumes added import when it is appreciated that this disability is becoming one of the most frequent causes of claims for compensation."

Lumbago is but a faint echo today. "I injured my back" is parlance, inside or outside the workplace. Hardly a physician elicits a history from a patient with regional backache without the query "What were you doing when it started?" Hardly a patient fails to volunteer the information when not asked. Attribution of regional backache to physical exposure is a social construction and, like osteopenia or fibromyalgia, it is now an *idée fixe* – a meme in some circles and "truth" in others. The fact that the attribution of back pain to a "ruptured disc" is scientifically untenable, as we saw in chapter 6, has done little to hamper the enormous surgical and non-surgical enterprises devoted to this idea. Because most of these "patients" are treated for regional back "injuries," much of this costly enterprise is underwritten by workers' compensation insurance, which indemnifies the medical care of these "injured" claimants.

This compensable back injury has been the rationale for a dramatic shift in the purview of industrial engineering. At mid-point in the twentieth century, ergonomics was the specialty in industrial engineering that analyzed the motion elements of industrial tasks so as to maximize performance. Ergonomics still retains this function, but, thanks to the pioneering efforts of Ernest Tischauer and, later, Stover Snook, maximizing worker comfort without sacrificing effectiveness became another goal. Tischauer incorporated biomechanics into the principles of tool and machine design. Snook's approach, termed psychophysics, was to explore the physical content and context of tasks in order to optimize worker acceptance. Soon another question arose concerning "injury." If a task was not designed according to the principles of biomechanics or of psychophysics, was it hazardous? Given the "injury" social construction, the affirmative answer made sense. Thousands of studies tried to define ergonomic hazards, studies notable for inconsistent outcomes and minor associations. Ergonomic advice flooded the industrial world, advice as to task design and safe biomechanics. The advice may still seem sensible, but it has never been shown to decrease the incidence of compensable backache. Still, social constructions die hard, and ergonomics keeps its political currency. The scientific refutation of the social construction that considers regional backache an "injury" is comprehensive, compelling, and reproducible. Whatever element of physical hazard outside of work, or ergonomic hazard in the modern workplace, is being missed must be so minor and so heterogeneous as to be irremediable.

We need to be very sceptical when someone touts any association between disabling regional musculoskeletal disorders and a wide range of physical exposures at work. Such associations can be detected, albeit inconsistently, in surveys where no alternative association is sought. However, nearly all multivariate cross-sectional and longitudinal studies of the association between disabling musculoskeletal disorders and either the psychosocial context of working or the physical demands of tasks find the former, generally to the exclusion of the latter. Because regional musculoskeletal disorders are intermittent and remittent predicaments of life, the likely explanation for these observations does not discount the symptoms, the morbidity. Episodes of backache, arm pain, and the like are the fate of all of us. When an episode is particularly daunting, we should direct our attention to the psychosocial context in which the morbidity plays out – a context that, when it confounds coping, renders the morbidity more memorable, less tolerable, and often disabling.

This dynamic is easily demonstrable outside the workplace, and the same principle pertains to backache at work. The worker with a backache has the option of seeking care for a back "injury," however, so long as all concerned agree that the backache arose out of, and in the course of, work. This care is indemnified by workers' compensation for the time it takes to reach maximum medical improvement, while income is also maintained. If "injured" workers have persistent work incapacity, they will not suffer any financial loss. Once they can prove disability, they will be compensated by workers' compensation insurance for lost wages. For the significant minority of American workers who have no health insurance and therefore no coverage for medical care for a backache, seeking care for a regional back "injury" is the only medical option. For others with health insurance, workers' compensation offers a far more advantaged form of recourse. Given these practical reasons, the ergonomic "injury" social construction is sacred to all labour advocates, even though the medical recourse and ergonomic interventions have been shown to be effete, useless, or even harmful.

Whenever a worker finds a regional musculoskeletal disorder disabling, the response should pivot on empathy, understanding, and community support. In all likelihood, it is a surrogate complaint indicating adverse aspects of the context of work that may be remedial. Medical recourse is ancillary. When a workforce is struck by an epidemic of disabling regional musculoskeletal disorders, the overwhelming probability is that there is an important lack in management style or in the architecture of work. Approaching such a circumstance under the "ergonomic injury" banner is likely to lead to two results: a cluster of workers bearing permanent scars from the quest for maximum medical improvement, and a workplace dripping ergonomic modifications to no demonstrable avail.

THE HAZARDS INHERENT IN AN ADVERSE PSYCHOSOCIAL CONTEXT OF WORKING

The frontier for epidemiology in this area is to further define "psychosocial context." That's an exercise that is nearly as daunting as defining the psychosocial correlates of poverty. Some of the common threads emerging from studies in the workplace include aspects of job "stress," "strain," "allostatic load," and motivational "flow." These measures are sampling such complex psychological functions as job satisfaction, perception of psychological demand, job autonomy, motivation, and the like. As such, associations with "psychosocial" variables are weak, even inconsistent. There may be much that is idiosyncratic. However, that variability does not diminish the implications; working in a psychosocial context that is adverse compromises coping with the next episode of a regional musculoskeletal disorder and places longevity at risk. The adverse psychosocial context may be peculiar to a particular worker who finds back pain disabling. There are also well-documented examples in large companies with multiple facilities of epidemics of disabling back or arm pain in a single facility. The physical demands of tasks are uniform across the facilities and are therefore not the culprit. Rather, the adverse context is peculiar to a particular facility. Usually, this situation is a reproach to management style in that facility.

The modern economy is providing us with another example of an idiosyncratic adverse context, where the adverse context relates to entire corporations or industries. The spectres of downsizing, outsourcing, or bankruptcy engulf the entire workforce in an adverse context rife with job insecurity and contentious personnel issues. The adverse health consequences for these workforces are considerable. A number of cohort studies render this point incontrovertible. In the early 1990s, for example, the Finnish economy suffered a considerable setback lasting several years. Many workers were dismissed. The effect of impending downsizing on the local government employees in one small city was monitored. The rate of absenteeism escalated, most markedly for sick leave ascribed to regional musculoskeletal disorders and particularly among employees over the age of fifty.

The "Whitehall" studies are cohort studies of British civil servants which documented an inverse relationship between civil service grade and mortality rate, particularly mortality from cardiovascular disease. In recent years it has become clear that the association with grade paled next to the association with psychosocial job "stress," especially job "control," regardless of grade. Similar relationships pertain to absence due to back pain.

One Whitehall cohort, faced with impending outsourcing, suffered a fate similar to that observed in the Finnish cohort. Impending downsizing wreaks havoc on the psychosocial context of work, inflicting "stress" and "strain" on all, particularly aging workers. Downsizing accelerates that noxious, insalubrious, and lethal process we are denoting as an adverse "psychosocial" work context. And it does so without regard for previous station in life.

Even without the inflammatory influences of downsizing, an adverse psychosocial context works its harm. Slowly it deprives individuals of favourable "self-rated health" (SRH). Like socioeconomic status, SRH is a powerful predictor of all-cause mortality. In a cohort of 5,001 Danish workers, adverse "psychosocial" work context was shown to erode SRH over the five years of observation. A similar association has emerged from analysis of Harvard's Nurses' Health Study; a perception that psychosocial work conditions were unfavourable predicted declining functional status among some 21,000 nurses followed for four years.

Several years ago, Wal-Mart and investigators from the National Institute of Occupational Health and Safety designed a cohort study to test whether wearing "back belts" prevented disabling back pain. It didn't. This large study followed some 6,000 employees in 160 stores for six months. At inception, volunteers were interviewed and queried extensively in an attempt to quantify their sense of psychological comfort at work. There was minimal discernible influence of the physical demands of tasks on the incidence of disabling back pain. However, the perception of high job-intensity demands and scheduling demands, as well as overall job dissatisfaction, were discernible as associating with the incidence of disabling back pain.

STRESS AND WELL-BEING

Stress is a difficult concept to define or grasp, probably because its meaning is largely dependent on context. "Stress" is not always bad.

Physical stress in biological systems has the same U-shaped cause-effect curve we discussed in chapter 2. For example, bone remodels to be stronger with a certain amount of physical stress. Furthermore, muscles are more effective, tendons stronger, and cartilage thicker. The ergonomic thrust aimed at banning physical stress from life, including life in the workplace, is a biologically flawed notion.

Psychological stress is not all bad either, nor can it be avoided. Psychological stress that leads to enhanced performance, which is satisfying and pleasing, is a goal in many aspects of vocational and avocational life. Learning how to overcome, or cope with, psychological stress is intrinsic to maturing and to assuming an effective role in the family and in society. Stress cannot be avoided, at least not for long. Attempting to avoid it is stressful.

In the workplace, safety can be regulated. Violent injuries are unconscionable, and all feasible efforts should be expended in enhancing safety so that accidents are rare. Can "stress" be regulated? How do you set up parameters of the context of work so that it is as stress free as possible, so that as many workers as possible feel "good in their skin" often or usually or always? Industrial psychologists can define work autonomy in a particular setting, but when they measure the association with job satisfaction, the variability is enormous, reflecting the differences among individuals. If there is to be any regulation of the psychosocial context of working, akin to regulations that abrogate hazards for physical harm, it would have to exhibit a broad tolerance for individual differences. There would have to be a level of awareness that elevated labour-management discourse and negotiation rather than mandatory standards of behaviour.

The humane solution is not in regulations. It resides in informing the body politic of the critical importance of the psychosocial context of work and in valuing workers, particularly those who have an innate talent in assisting co-workers to cope effectively with stress. These caring leaders are invaluable. The modern workplace offers an important opportunity to help those who are lacking in the wherewithal to improve their self-esteem, their coping skills, and their longevity.

None of this ideal will come to pass until the social constructions relating to "injury," to "in your mind," and to "human capital" are superseded. Today men and women are choosing to be patients and claimants because their ability to cope with their regional musculoskeletal disorder is inadequate to the challenge of maintaining their self-respect in the adverse context of their employment. In responding to their charge to mitigate their dilemma, the occupational health establishment must learn that anatomical conditions do not delineate their illness. Just as we have learned that impediments to coping beleaguer patients with rheumatoid arthritis and the elderly with knee pain, so society must broach discussions of life in the workplace for the sake of these patients. Doctors may be as powerless as patients to put things right, or, perhaps, some solution may emerge. A solution becomes more likely if we gain expertise in the dynamics of the workplace and identify resources that can assist us, much as we have regarding life in the home. Society should bridle whenever "human capital" is held up as expendable.

10

Why Are Alternative and Complementary Therapies Thriving?

Alternative therapies are a controversial topic, one that challenges the objectivity of all health-care professionals. I shall use them as an opportunity to revisit the themes of this book from a different slant. To begin, I'll be open about my own prejudices.

- I am convinced that complementary and alternative therapies thrive best whenever my guild, which requires an MD for admission, is behaving in an unconscionable manner.
- I can countenance no treatment modality or treatment act that has an unfavourable benefit/risk ratio, regardless of the purveyor.
- I am willing to share the cost for someone to query whether the benefit/risk ratio of any therapeutic modality or treatment act is favourable.
- I am willing to share the cost of the therapeutic modality if the benefit/risk ratio is favourable.
- For treatment acts that some find beneficial, yet are based on modalities that are neither harmful nor beneficial, I reserve the option of refusing to share the cost.
- However, I bridle at having to share the cost of underwriting any therapeutic envelope.

These assertions are anything but straightforward. Defining them, let alone serving them, takes science to its limits. Even with definitional licence, the ramifications are considerable.

That will become clear in the discussions that follow: a brief history of complementary and alternative therapy; the concept of moral hazard; and the notions of treatment modality, treatment act, and therapeutic envelope.

A BRIEF HISTORY OF COMPLEMENTARY AND ALTERNATIVE THERAPY

The ancient Egyptians prayed to Imhotep. The Romans borrowed the Greek demigod Asclepios. Aesculapius was a son of Apollo who begot two sons – Machaon, the surgeon, and Podalirios, the physician – and two daughters, Hygieia and Panacea. For the ancients, gods and demigods could cause and cure diseases and wounds. Healing gods were enshrined in special temples open to all who were ill and suffering. Physicians were itinerant crafts-men, ministering and operating in the homes of those who could pay their fee. Mythology began to give way to scientific medicine thanks to Hippocrates, who was born on the island of Cos about 460 BCE. On his death at the age of eighty, he left a legacy shrewd in clinical observations and ethical commentaries that have held theological and superstitious clinical theories and practices somewhat at bay ever since. Hippocrates' clinical observations were complemented by the theories of his contem-porary, Plato, to spawn the Dogmatists' school of medicine. For this group, observation was a poor substitute for reasoning. Many vitalistic theories, self-determining forces beyond the prin-ciples of biology, spewed forth as the rationale for extreme ther-apeutic measures, including purging, bleeding, and dehydrating the ill. The history of medicine ever since has involved the dis-carding of vitalistic theories in favour of those that are scientif-ically tenable, and the fashioning of remedies that bridle therapeutic zeal with requirements for evidence of effectiveness. In spite of all the intervening centuries of progress, much about illness remains beyond the reach of tested theories, as does much therapeutic zeal.

The history of care for the ill and the history of medicine are parallel, but not monolithic. Many around the globe who are ill still seek refuge in superstition and theology, some by choice and some by default. Furthermore, there are, and always have been, purveyors of remedies that are beyond the reach of testing, often based on theories that defy contemporary reasoning and earn the scorn of the modern Dogmatists. Others earn the scorn of scientific medicine. Scorned or not, treatments of all varieties flourish. Some predate my guild. Some that are only a century or two old remain active participants in the Western health-care delivery scene today. In the resource-challenged world, alternatives to my guild often predominate. In fact, it is only in the past century that Western medicine has managed to secure its position on the pinnacle.

A millennium ago, Europe sacrificed its intellectual roots and traditions to superstition and lapsed into the Dark Ages. Meanwhile, science, philosophy, and medicine thrived in the Arab world, with centres of excellence such as Alexandria. Japanese and Chinese medicine and medical education also advanced in rationality and organization. The Western resurgence began with William Harvey's observation on the circulation of blood. It made slow progress through the eighteenth century in terms of theory, some progress in terms of surgery, but painfully slow progress in medical treatment (therapeusis). Purging, bleeding, and other forms of therapeutic violence predominated, the legacy of the Dogmatists.

At the turn of the nineteenth century, Samuel Hahnemann, a German physician, offered an alternative approach to treatment. He had turned to experimental pharmacology, looking for agents with greater benefit/risk ratios than those in common use. He tested substances on himself and his family, beginning with Jesuit's bark (see chapter 6), experiments he termed "drug provings." He developed his theory of "similia similibus"; if a drug produced symptoms in a well person, then very small doses (the "law of infinitesimals") would cure similar symptoms in someone who was ill. He named his system of therapeusis "homeopathy" and termed the standard practice of mainstream physicians "allopathy." Allopathic physicians, he argued, administered drugs that counter the symptoms of illness (then conceptualized as the disease) – for instance, an antipyretic for fever. He advocated administering tiny doses of a drug that could cause fever in high doses. Some people still label doctors in my guild "allopathic physicians," but I find the term unacceptable, since so much that we offer is no longer symptomatic treatment (antibiotics, for example).

Homeopathy proved very successful in recruiting patients, practitioners, and advocates in Europe and in North America. In 1842 Oliver Wendell Holmes, then dean of the Harvard Medical School, delivered two lectures entitled "Homeopathy and Its Kindred Delusions," in which he warned against "fatal credulity" in any of the alternatives then claiming "wonderful powers." Here we have the greatest mind in medicine of his generation casting aspersions as a spokesman for a profession that was still bleeding and purging. Homeopathy was unfazed. Indeed, it remained so successful that it challenged the dominance of the traditional medical guild in the American market. At the turn of the twentieth century, organized medicine capitulated and assimilated the homeopaths and their educational institutions (the Hahnemann Medical School in Philadelphia, and the Flower Fifth Avenue School in New York City, now the New York Medical College in Valhalla). Homeopathy remains an alternative system of therapeusis in much of the Western world to this day, and it is enjoying resurgence in North America.

A contemporary of Hahnemann, Franz Anton Mesmer, became a celebrity because of his theories of "animal magnetism." His Magnetic Institute in Paris attracted the somatizing rich, particularly young female somatizing rich, until he and his followers were banished to Switzerland for operating beyond the bounds of the moral propriety of the day. Mesmer left two legacies, hypnotic suggestion (hence the verb "to mesmerize") and the notion of magnetism. Therapeutic magnets are enjoying such resurgence today that the prestigious *Journal of the American Medical Association* felt it appropriate to publish a study that fails to discern any therapeutic benefit from them. Across the channel from Mesmer and Hahnemann, Dr James Graham operated his Temple of Health and Hygiene in London. Graham is remembered more for his therapeutic diet, particularly his therapeutic cracker, than for medicalizing moral turpitude in a fashion that rivalled Mesmer. While all this was happening, Edward Jenner discovered vaccination.

In the eighteenth century only the wealthy could afford to partake of the wonders of modern medicine, though these wonders hardly had much to recommend them. The masses made do on their own or turned to the apothecaries, who functioned as the primary care practitioners of the day. All sorts of potions were purveyed. The nineteenth century may have witnessed the birth of modern scientific medicine, though that advance was much more in terms of theory than practice. For mainstream practitioners, this century was one of "heroic medicine." Therapeutic zeal seemed to recognize no treatment boundaries. Bleeding, purging, and fever therapies, along with administering heavy metals and toxic botanical potions and unctions, were the order of the day. "Heroic medicine" was a term that grew out of the carnage on the battlefields and in the military hospitals of the Civil War and entered civilian life.

Not surprisingly, society welcomed old remedies and invented new alternatives. Homeopaths claimed recovery rates in the cholera epidemic of 1849 that outstripped the track record of mainstream ministrations. A century would elapse before epidemiology began to contend with confounders and bias in such observations, so there is considerable uncertainty about these claims. Perhaps the sicker patients chose mainstream physicians, or perhaps the mainstream ministrations ushered more to their deaths. Regardless, it was sensible to seek alternatives when ill. The nineteenth-century menu of alternatives was extensive. There were schools of hydrotherapists and botanical therapists. North America's answer to Graham's dietary-plus approach to wellness was thriving in Michigan, where Dr Will Kellogg offered hydrotherapy, colonic irrigation, purging, abdominal surgery, and clitoral stimulation along with his therapeutic corn flakes. In response to "heroic medicine" and all the quackery, the nineteenth century birthed a religious backlash that included Christian Science and the Pentecostal movement.

Homeopathy and other therapeutic movements that challenge the tenets of mainstream medicine are termed "sectarian" by my guild. "Sectarian medicine" is a pejorative term. It is not meant to imply that all sectarian practitioners are cultists or even true believers; rather, it designates the systems of health care that compete both with each other and with mainstream medicine. All are capable of taking off their gloves to protect their turf. They seek licensure as a public acknowledgment of the specialized nature of their knowledge and skills, as well as to codify a competitive advantage in that regard. They are perhaps more akin to guilds of old than to present-day unions. All compete for "the health-care dollar." Like other businesses, some flourish, some merge, and many fold. Homeopathy in the United States is one that merged, disappearing into mainstream medicine for many decades, though it appears to be rising anew. Others maintain a life of their own. Two made-in-America examples of sectarian medicine are worthy of our attention: osteopathy and the chiropractic.

As a young man, Andrew Taylor Still (1828–1917) was apprenticed to a physician. He became disillusioned with medical practice when he witnessed the heroic measures undertaken by the physicians attending his three children as they succumbed to meningitis in the epidemic in 1864. The son of a Methodist minister, Still believed that imbibing alcohol was sinful. If alcohol was sinful, other drugs must be too. He was drawn to the theories of Mesmer and the magnetic healers, with their belief that diseases were caused by interruptions in the pathways for magnetic fluids in the body. The magnetic healers used magnets to redirect that flow. Instead of magnets, Still postulated that the manipulative techniques (long practised by bonesetters and the like) would work as well as magnets, if not better. He founded his school of osteopathy in Kirksville, Missouri, teaching others how to "realign displacements" – obstructing musculoskeletal segments usually in the spine. Once realigned, natural healing could proceed without recourse to allopathic drugs. By the turn of the twentieth century, Still had an infirmary in Kirksville, over seven hundred graduates, and a sizable following.

Osteopathic schools opened elsewhere. Patients who were under the care of osteopaths fared better than those treated to "heroic medicine" in the influenza epidemic of 1918–19, harkening back to homeopaths' claims in the 1849 cholera epidemic. Over the objections of Still, then eighty-seven years old, the American Osteopathic Association decided to incorporate the "materia medica" of mainstream medicine into the curriculum in the early twentieth century. By the middle of the century, there were fifteen schools of osteopathic medicine, with curricula similar to that of the traditional medical schools. By the 1960s all states licensed osteopaths with privileges comparable to those of MDs. Nonetheless, the American Osteopathic Association maintains control over accreditation of these schools, grants a DO degree, and mandates courses in musculoskeletal manipulation, although the vitalistic theories that seduced Still are long gone. Michigan State University houses curricula leading to either the MD or the DO degree in the same facility and sharing courses in common.

The chiropractic and mainstream medicine have no such cozy relationship. The chiropractic was founded in the Midwest in 1895, in Davenport, Iowa, by Daniel David Palmer (1845–1913). Palmer was a grocer who, like Still, was into vitalism. He reasoned that excessive "tone" produced "impingement, a pressure on nerves," from which disease resulted. "Adjusting vertebrae, using the spinous and transverse processes as lever," could relieve that "tone." Palmer claimed to have cured a janitor of deafness and said he could improve the condition of patients with heart failure – all by manipulation of the neck. By the turn of the twentieth century, Palmer had a school, an infirmary, students, and a moniker for his sectarian therapy. The name, chiropractic, is derived from the Greek *cheir* (hand) and *praxis* (specific use). His son, B.J. Palmer, was one of his first students and, later, he purchased the school and managed to turn it into a successful enterprise. Palmer Jr and his followers were proponents of pure, "straight," unadulterated chiropractic. However, this example of sectarian medicine soon turned sectarian within itself. "Mixers" were willing to incorporate the practices of other sects into their own: "napropaths," who treated irritated ligaments instead of impinged nerves; "neuropaths," who felt the impingements were outside the spine; and others such as physiotherapists and naturopaths, who developed from botanists and herbalists. Several of these splinter sects have faded away, but not all, and several are making a comeback. To this day a schism persists in the chiropractic between "mixers" and "straights," particularly "straight-straights," who adhere to D.D. Palmer's vitalistic theory.

The bickering within the chiropractic pales next to the open warfare with the medical establishment that played out through much of the twentieth century. By mid-point, the American Medical Association held the chiropractic to be quackery and declared interactions with chiropractors on a professional level to be unethical. The battle moved into the marketplace, where the chiropractic thrives and practitioners now number around 60,000, mainly in the United States. It also moved into the courts, so that by 1975 the chiropractic was licensed in all states and, four years later, the formalized prejudice of the American Medical Association was found to be illegal. "Straights" or "mixers," chiropractors are licensed to perform manipulative therapies and imaging studies, but not to prescribe pharmaceuticals.

What is less defined, somewhat contentious within the chiropractic, and very contentious for mainstream medicine is the purview of the chiropractic. Is it solely the regional musculoskeletal disorders? That is not the stance of many chiropractors or many schools of chiropractic. These advocates and practitioners are willing to "reduce subluxations" for a range of ailments from headache to asthma. Subluxations are the chiropractic diagnosis that implies spinal malalignment. They are imaginary; no such specific skeletal changes correlate with symptoms. However, chiropractors are skilled at applying a brief, high-velocity force to the vertebral column sufficient to create a vacuum phenomenon in the small joints of the spine. The vacuum phenomenon snaps back with cracking sounds and sensations, which cause the chiropractor to feel accomplished and the patient to feel treated. How anyone can imagine that such an event can salve asthma or diabetes or the like is a testimony to the tenacity of vitalistic theories.

Turning the cracking of backs and necks into a fastidious art form is the triumph of the chiropractic. These manœuvres take their place in the ancient tradition of manual therapy. Therapeutic massage can be traced back through history. Medical luminaries of their day employed and wrote about massage, traction, and manipulation: Avicenna in the eleventh century, Charef-Ed-Din in the fifteenth century, and Ambroise Paré in the sixteenth century are but a few. Manipulation of the skeleton is mainstream in osteopathy, where the manipulation traditionally entails the application of shearing force using less acceleration and generally a longer lever arm than the chiropractic. It is central to the system of "orthopaedic medicine" formulated by James Cyriax in London thirty years ago, and to the physiotherapy school of Robert Maigne that is commonly practised in Europe. Manual therapy is part of the fabric of life today, in all cultures, and always will be.

I am a rheumatologist, a mainstream physician with an MD, schooled in and committed to the care of patients with musculoskeletal disorders. Do I have to learn manual medicine? Should I seek such a salve for my own next predicament of a regional musculoskeletal disorder? Should I refer my patients to such practitioners?

There are corollary issues. Should I encourage or applaud recourse to the morass of putative neutriceuticals, herbal and botanical remedies, dietary supplements, and the like? There are professionals who claim skills in the purveyance of these remedies, including naturopaths and homeopaths. Does their ministration benefit their patients? As we discussed in chapter 6, mainstream physicians were all herbalists till quite recently. Herbal remedies, botanicals, and other naturally occurring organic and inorganic substances were all that was available before the twentieth century, and they remained the mainstream physician's stock in trade until the last half of that century. Frankincense and myrrh were expectorants and astringents, for instance, as well as ecclesiastical accoutrements. The advances of the last half of that century include the ability to purify and synthesize pharmacologically active compounds, the ability to establish dose-response curves, and the mandate to assess benefit/risk ratios.

Do you really think there is something important being overlooked among the folk remedies or the formulations of naturopaths and homeopaths? Maybe you are right in such thinking. Maybe the pharmaceutical industry is so interested in profit margins that substances which cannot be patented are left undeveloped. Certainly there are botanicals with pharmacological effects yet to be discovered, and more certainly biologicals with pharmacological effects yet to be purified. But there are none that should circumvent the benefit/risk gantlet to marketing. We should not forgo the assessment of benefit/risk ratios just because these substances are naturally occurring. Some may be harmful or have tight therapeutic ratios, the margin between effect and toxicity. That's true for some of the classic botanicals, such as digitalis and colchicines, which are still in use (though in pure form). Digitalis was isolated from the foxglove and is still used for some cardiac disorders, even though the line between benefit and fatal toxicity is very fine. With colchicine, still used to prevent gouty attacks, the fine line is between benefit and diarrhea.

To address these queries, we need to visit the difficult issue of health insurance. There are many purveyors of many remedies. What is covered? What is not? Can we infer a favourable benefit/risk ratio for those remedies that are covered by insurance?

MORAL HAZARDS

At the turn of the twentieth century, few Westerners were insured for anything. There were burial societies, such as the Friendly Societies in Britain, which offered the worker who could afford to join one the peace of mind that his family, probably left bereft of support by his death, would not be further burdened by his funeral expenses. But insurance was largely unavailable – and not because it was unheard of. To the contrary, indemnity was a pressing political issue in Victorian times. There was no debate that there are hazards that cannot be wholly avoided and that are catastrophic for any single victim unless the impact is blunted by sharing the fiscal consequences with others at risk. There was no doubt that indemnity schemes could offer a solution to this human predicament. The debate that raged then, and will not be stilled, relates to "moral hazard." Just as a homeowner who needs money can burn down his house and try to claim the insurance, will a worker claim disability as a reflection of job dissatisfaction or insecurity rather than work incapacity? How can anyone police such behaviour?

Property insurance set the precedent with investigations and inflated premiums to compensate for stealth immorality. Personal injury and the rest of social insurance followed in a dialectic that knows no closure. Its history is grounded in the Prussian "welfare monarchy," which was fathered by Bismarck and rapidly adopted by Lloyd George and the rest of the industrialized world early in the twentieth century. When Bismarck was finished, Prussia had a national health insurance scheme and a stratified disability scheme. The debate on the latter was heated, relating to the moral hazard inherent in choosing to be a disability claimant. Even Wilbur Cohen, when he was crafting the Social Security Disability scheme in the United States at mid-century, had to contend with the moral hazard argument. It is traditional to frame moral hazard as a failing of the claimant and to seek administrative remedies in light of this problem. In chapter 9 we touched on the price paid by any claimant who is drawn into the Kafkaesque experience of having to prove illness. But little has been said of the other moral hazards that lurk in the personal injury and disability indemnity schemes.

Indemnity schemes carry their own constituencies. If they are publicly held, the constituency is made up of administrators and supportive politicians. If they are private enterprises, the constituency is the administrators and the stakeholders. Premiums will diminish if claims are reduced or if their processing is more efficient. In that case the size of the enterprise and the power of its administrators will diminish as well, usually dragging down their compensation and the profits paid to stockholders. There is a moral hazard in the drive to maintain the size, scope, and profitability of the insurance enterprise, a danger that is bounded on one side by the social constructions that relate to what needs to be covered and how much it should cost, and on the other side by the ability of the insured to afford putatively adequate coverage. There is no better illustration than the "health" insurance industry in the United States.

Health insurance underwrites the entire enterprise that occupied our attention in Part One of this book. Among those who have insurance, the Last Well Person is faced with the task of discerning the interventions that are readily available and administered expertly but that advantage them not at all. The plight of the 30 million Americans without health insurance does not relate simply to the inaccessibility of effective remedies in the short run, but to the toll that their socioeconomic status will mete out to them and their families in the long run. Health insurers and workers' compensation insurers divvy up the business relating to the regional musculoskeletal disorders based on the "injury" semantic, as we saw in chapters 6 and 9. However, it is only recently that health and workers' compensation insurers have been "pressed" to indemnify sectarian care.

Once the chiropractic successfully challenged its ostracism by the American Medical Association, the argument followed that workers with disabling regional musculoskeletal "injuries" should have the choice of ministrations. After all, the patient population of the chiropractic was enriched for individuals with regional musculoskeletal disorders, even for those with indemnified musculoskeletal injuries consequent to motor vehicle accidents. Should the chiropractic be excluded from providing care for "injured" workers whose workers' compensation insurance entitled them to all types of care to make them as well as possible? And should chiropractors be excluded from providing care for musculoskeletal injuries resulting from motor vehicle accidents? Today, the worker with a regional back "injury" is likely to be both scarred by a surgeon and making frequent visits to a chiropractor. Once the health insurance industry began underwriting chiropractic care, patients with backache who turned to chiropractors were likely to return more frequently, for longer periods, and with greater satisfaction than if they had chosen to see either a primary care physician or an orthopaedist. There is no difference in cost between these categories of providers because the frequency of visits to chiropractors compensates for their relatively reduced costliness. The chiropractic has managed a political and legal campaign that has gained its practitioners provider status for musculoskeletal disorders on nearly all forms of health insurance except that afforded by the Veterans Administration.

Meanwhile, health-care and workers' compensation premiums escalate. Where is the value?

COMPLEMENTARY AND ALTERNATIVE MODALITIES, TREATMENT ACTS, AND THERAPEUTIC ENVELOPES

Modalities are what are done for us, to us, or with us by any purveyor of therapy to whom we turn. The treatment act acknowledges that modalities seldom operate without human interaction with their purveyor. The context in which the modalities are offered and administered is the treatment act. It's the whole process of intervention of the provider on behalf of the patient. The therapeutic envelope refers to the way in which we are changed by the treatment act. It is our new being, the sum of our altered self-perception, idiom of distress, narrative of illness, and peer affinities, as well as our expectations for our healthfulness and from our community. Entering into a treatment envelope is entering into another station in life, never to return, often, regardless of the clinical outcome. The Last Well Person is aware, before initiating the process, of both the potential far-reaching personal impact of accepting treatment and the effectiveness of the various modalities. No one should enter a therapeutic envelope without awareness of the passage and the acceptance of the outcome.

Over-the-Counter Modalities

Some modalities seem free of a treatment act, let alone a therapeutic envelope, because no professional person is directly involved in their purveyance. That's a false impression. The choice to purchase a putative neutraceutical, botanical, or other dietary supplement is always informed. These substances are frequently mentioned in the lay medical press and are aggressively marketed. Wherever you make your purchase, you will have access to "informed" and helpful salespeople. There is a community to welcome you, a community of believers who feel advantaged in some way by participating in this sectarian treatment act. You will either join their therapeutic domain or not. There is no middle ground.

There also is no attempt to provide any assurance of purity, safety, or efficacy. That is a policy decision: the *Dietary Supplement and Health Education Act* of 1994 permits the unregulated sale of herbal and other botanical products that were already on the shelf. The argument held that such substances are foodstuffs, not pharmaceuticals. The burden of proof of safety and purity resides with the manufacturer, who may describe physiological effects and imply benefits but may not promote effectiveness. As for purity, many studies demonstrate the enormous variability in the constituents marketed as the same substance by different manufacturers. One study of Asian patent medicines sold in California in 1998 showed that a third of these so-called botanicals were adulterated with undeclared pharmaceuticals or heavy metals that were biologically active and potentially toxic: ephedrine, chlorpheniramine, methyltestosterone, phenacetin, lead, mercury, and arsenic were detected. Believers in, and purveyors of, herbal preparations find refuge from critics in the sheer variability in the ingredients of the manufactured preparations, as well as in the number of patent preparations sold by vendors. They claim that their preparation is different from the preparation that fared poorly in the latest randomized controlled trial. There is no rational counter-argument, nor is there a feasible way to study everyone's pet remedy.

Even apart from these undesirable contaminants, herbs themselves, like conventional pharmaceuticals, can have unexpected side effects – effects that are not systematically screened for. Any adverse effects, if they are reported at all, will be detected only in the post-marketing arena. Even with this haphazard surveillance,

Table 10.1
Possible Adverse Effects of Some Herbal Products

Herbal Product	Adverse Effect
Chaparral, Comfrey, Germander	Liver disease
Slimming tea	Nausea and vomiting ... possible death
Jin Bu Huan	Depressed heart, mind, lung function
Lobelia	Coma and death at high dose
Yohimbe	Kidney disease, seizures and death

the FDA has identified toxicities, as set out in a partial listing in table 10.1.

Chaso and Onshido belong on the list. These Chinese herbal weight-loss aids are widely available over the Internet and have become popular in Japan. They are effective in inducing weight loss only when they cause acute and severe liver damage. Ephedra also belongs on the list, particularly as it is included in a number of "diet" preparations. It is also called Ma Huang and epitonin. Its benefit/risk ratio is very small, and its adverse effects on the cardiovascular and central nervous system are well documented. Various authorities, including Sid Wolfe of the Public Citizen Health Research Group, urged the FDA to ban this agent and finally prevailed in the winter of 2004. The purveyors had argued that too few people are harmed for there to be any concern, but the product has such marginal effectiveness that any toxicity is unconscionable.

There is another, growing list of dietary supplements that can disturb the effectiveness of licensed pharmaceuticals. Some increase and others inhibit the effects of conventional drugs, just as some foodstuffs do – rhubarb and grapefruit, for example. As more drug-food interactions are uncovered, physicians and pharmacists are trained to alert their patients. Who is there to forewarn the consumer about potential interactions between usual foodstuffs and putatively therapeutic "dietary supplements"?

I am not convinced that anything on the health-food shelf has a worthy benefit/risk ratio. Ginkgo is of questionable use for dementia. St John's Wort shows little benefit as an anti-depressant and offers considerable concerns about interactions with licensed drugs. Ginseng and echinacea are expensive, and clinical trials have failed to discern any advantage in them, in particular in ginseng for dementia and in echinacea for the common cold. Saw palmetto may do something if you have prostatism, but it also may not. Phytoestrogen supplements do not banish hot flashes, and guggulipids will not reduce your serum cholesterol. Even though there are herbal remedies and dietary supplements that may do some good, they all have downsides. As far as I'm concerned, they are all worthless unless they taste good.

That is not the "word on the street," however, or the word in advertising. Companies can market herbal remedies and other dietary supplements without approval of the FDA or any other regulatory agency. The Internet, in particular, holds many examples of egregious marketing practices. Even when controlled by the FDA and other agencies, advertisers often play fast and loose with the truth. The editor of the *New England Journal of Medicine* has, on occasion, felt compelled to decry the licence taken by advertisers with science published in his journal. A systematic review of the content of advertisements in leading medical journals performed several years ago documents the plethora of assertions that outside experts find misleading. The uninformed person is at a disadvantage in the marketing arena and will be well served by scepticism when faced with claims about dietary supplements. For that matter, the Last Well Person should also be sceptical about the claims of licensed pharmaceuticals in direct-to-consumer marketing, whether by celebrities on television or in convoluted prose in the print media. I suggest you close your eyes when the next televised advertisement for a prescription drug appears. Listen to the convoluted and obfuscating prose without being distracted by someone on ice skates, or a football coach, or whatever. As for print media, have someone else read the prose to you so you won't see the pictures. These exercises will do wonders for your scepticism.

Then there are the vitamins. A recent study from Britain suggests that taking a single (large) dose of vitamin D once every four months will reduce the incidence of vertebral fractures as effectively as any bisphosphonate. Britain lacks sunlight in certain months of the year. Since sun exposure releases endogenous vitamin D, the observation in Britain may not pertain to sunnier climes. However, the cohort in this study was elderly, aged sixty-five to eighty-five at inception, and the observation may well pertain to elderly cohorts in other parts of the world. There cannot be many other subsets of well people in the resource-advantaged world who are vitamin deficient. Public health regulations ensure that foods are supplemented with vitamins to guard against any such deficiency. If you are well, well nourished, and not unusual in your dietary proclivities, you are not vitamin deficient. Yet it is estimated that a third of the US population uses vitamin supplements regularly – a testimony to marketing and the preconceived notions of the lay medical press. The issue for us is whether the lay press is prescient.

There is one special but unequivocal affirmative to this question. The daily recommended intake of folic acid is too little in the first trimester of pregnancy. With further supplementation, the likelihood of neural tube defects (spina bifida and the like) is reduced significantly. Are there other examples, other subsets of the well and the well-nourished that would be advantaged in some clinically meaningful way by vitamin supplements? The lay health press and the industry that purveys vitamin supplements have conspired to render it an urgent matter. Large and expensive trials have been undertaken and more are under way. There is no shortcut to testing whether a vitamin supplement will lead to a subtle advantage or disadvantage other than a large and long-term randomized controlled trial. We can only wonder whether such a subtle health effect is worth so much effort, or whether any subtle effect that is discerned will be convincing, reliable, or even meaningful.

Some of the most compelling effects to emerge from these trials are negative. Take the carotenoids, for example. There are hundreds of carotenoids; all are antioxidants, and many have pro-vitamin A activity – meaning they are converted in the body to retinol, the active vitamin necessary for normal vision and other functions. It has long been known that individuals can ingest too much vitamin A, leading to skin and liver disease. However, the doses recommended by those who think the daily recommendation inadequate fall far short of these toxic doses. Antioxidants in general and carotenoids in particular are thought by some to have the potential to prevent a variety of degenerative diseases. Carotenoids have been formally studied in cohort and randomized controlled trials to see if they prevent emphysema, coronary artery disease, or prostate cancer. No consistent benefit has been discerned. However, for individuals who abuse tobacco and take carotenoids, their risk of lung cancer is increased. Furthermore, supplements have been shown to increase the risk of fractures, so much so that some researchers are wondering if the recommended daily intake is too much. The US Preventive Services Task Force has stated that, while some observational studies were encouraging, all randomized controlled trials of vitamin supplementation to stave off cancer or cardiovascular disease have proved disappointing.

Vitamin E is another antioxidant. Among the several randomized controlled trials in coronary artery disease that have included this vitamin, most discern no effect at all, and none discern an effect on mortality. The most impressive trial, the Heart Outcomes Prevention Evaluation (HOPE) study, randomized almost 10,000 patients at risk for cardiovascular events because they had previous events and because the prevalence of the "metabolic syndrome" in this group was high. Treatment with vitamin E for 4.5 years had no discernible clinical effect on cardiac outcomes, nor was there a discernible effect of vitamin E supplementation for the risk for stroke or respiratory tract infections.

Vitamin E supplementation may, however, diminish the likelihood of dementia. The Rotterdam study is a cohort study, not a drug trial. Over 5,000 older people have now been followed for an average of six years. Careful dietary histories, emphasizing antioxidant consumption, have been collected both at inception and at intervals ever since. Two hundred of these people developed some cognitive deficiency, of which 150 qualified as Alzheimer's disease. Those with cognitive deficiencies were more likely to have avoided high intake of vitamins E and C. Vitamin E has emerged, barely, as beneficial in decreasing the likelihood of dementia in two other cohort studies. Vitamin C and other antioxidants remain in the rumour category.

We should return to folic acid. It has been shown that an elevated plasma homocysteine level associates with coronary artery disease (as do many other things). It is also known that folic acid supplementation reduces that level. Several large randomized clinical trials are currently under way on folic acid supplementation. One trial, the Swiss Heart Study, suggests that lowering the homocysteine level with folic acid and vitamins B_6 and B_{12} decreases the complications of angioplasty for coronary artery disease. Folic acid supplementation of flour has been practised in the United States only since 1996. Before that, uncooked leafy vegetables, whole-grain cereals, and animal products were the richest natural sources. Maybe the new policy (initiated because of the spina bifida experience) is doing much more good beyond pregnancy. Longevity continues to increase, but there are better explanations than folic acid in our bread.

Hands-on Modalities

According to a recent telephone survey of some 2,000 randomly selected homes, about a third of adult Americans recall back or neck pain during the previous year. Of these, a third participated in complementary treatment acts; a third sought care from a member of my guild; and a quarter played safe and used both. Fuelled by social constructions and the broadening of coverage by Health Maintenance Organizations (HMOs) and other health insurers, the trend to seeing both physician and non-physician practitioners has escalated in the past decade. It is not clear whether seeing both represents an increase in conjoint service delivery or fragmentation of care. I suspect the latter. It is not clear how often physicians are aware that their patient is being attended simultaneously by a non-physician clinician or how often a physician coordinates treatment acts with the non-physician or confronts the cognitive dissonance of the different therapeutic envelopes. I suspect patients fend for themselves in

Table 10.2
Therapeutic Recourse Chosen by Americans for Their Backache

Modality	Treatment Act	% Using
Physical		35
	Chiropractic	20
	Massage	14
	Yoga	2
	Acupuncture	1
	Osteopathy	0.3
Digestives		5
	Homeopathy	3
	Vitamins	2
	Herbs	1
	Naturopathy	0
Cognitive		17
	Relaxation techniques	11
	Imagery	6
	Biofeedback	0.5
	Self-help	0.3
	Hypnosis	0
Other		16
	Spiritual healing	5
	Energy healing	4
	Aromatherapy	3
	Neural therapy	2
	Special diet	1
	Other	2

this regard. Table 10.2 sets out the relative choices from the menu of health-care alternatives.

For the 10 per cent of adult Americans who turn to alternative providers instead of, or in addition to, members of my guild, physical modalities have the greatest appeal. In this survey, the three most commonly purchased treatments were chiropractic, massage, and relaxation techniques. The treatments were rated as "very helpful" by 61 per cent, 65 per cent, and 43 per cent, respectively, by the people participating in these treatment acts, whereas only 27 per cent of patients attending a member of my guild found their treatment act "very helpful." Before you leap to the conclusion that the increased satisfaction expressed by those treated by non-physicians is a reflection of the modality, you should examine the "complementary" studies discussed below.

Another survey of American adults who chose alternative therapies demonstrated that they were predominately white, married, middle aged, and educated; had less robust self-reported health status; and described the alternative treatment acts as more congruent with their own values, beliefs, and philosophical orientations towards health and life. This finding was borne out in a survey of chiropractic patients, with the additional insight that their self-reported "mental health" was as worrisome as their self-reported general health status. Taken together, these observations are consonant with those I discussed in chapter 6. Life challenges that impair coping are an incentive to seek treatment for physical illness, and the treatment act offered by my guild is unsatisfactory compared with that offered by some of the others. Also, the more satisfying alternatives require, or provoke, agreement between the provider and the recipient about belief in the efficacy of the particular healing system. The 10 per cent of Americans identified in the tabulation above are comfortably ensconced in a therapeutic envelope, which requires their sharing the belief system on which the alternative treatment act is grounded. Is this sophistry – therapeutic, but sophistry nonetheless? To be effective, any treatment act must consider the preconceived notions that the patient carries to the encounter. These belief systems are part of the persona of the patient, and they influence participation in the treatment act and its outcome. Value judgments have little place in this consideration. However, to turn belief systems into therapeutic tools is to walk a fine line between the ranks of the clerics and the ranks of the charlatans.

A wealth of science tests the effectiveness of the physical modalities listed above, as well as some not listed. The effectiveness of particular modalities is fundamental to the various therapeutic belief systems in such a way that tests of the effectiveness of a modality are viewed as a test of the credibility of the treatment act. So many randomized controlled trials of various forms of massage and spinal manipulation for regional back and neck pain have been reported that there are not just systematic reviews and meta-analyses, but systematic reviews and meta-analyses of the systematic reviews. These reports are studies of modalities, of particular forms of the "laying on of hands." With one exception, there is no compelling or even suggestive evidence that any of the physical modalities in table 10.2 offers any discernible benefit. A similar conclusion pertains to trials of acupuncture, physical therapy, and massage. There are even randomized controlled trials of "therapeutic touch" and "distant healing," and they yield little encouragement – if any.

The one exception relates to spinal manipulation. In 1987 my colleagues and I published a randomized controlled trial we had performed with funding from the Robert Wood Johnson Foundation. We recruited from the community young people who had been suffering from acute regional back pain for less than a month, who had never undergone any form of spinal manipulation in the past, and whose predicament was not confounded by issues of work incapacity. All the recruits were examined by me and reassured. All underwent a mobilization – they were gently moved from side to side and treated with flexion/extension by my colleague and co-investigator, a professor of family medicine who had been trained by James Cyriax in London in "orthopaedic medicine." Half of them underwent a long-lever arm, high-velocity, lateral-thrust "back crack" – the basic manœuvre of osteopathy. All the subjects felt better as they left the office, regardless of the procedure. For those who had been hurting for two weeks or less at the time of the intervention, all were better two weeks later, and the pace of healing was not influenced by the modality. For those who had been hurting for two to four weeks at the time of the intervention, all were better two weeks later, but those who received the single "back crack" healed more rapidly.

The world of spinal manipulation holds this investigation up as a landmark, and the result has been reproduced many times. However, it does not reproduce in any other subset of people suffering back pain. Only those who have had non-confounded regional backache for two to four weeks benefit from spinal manipulation, and then only from a single encounter. Furthermore, the benefit is measured only in days of extra relief, not more.

All these studies attempt to test a therapeutic modality independent of the treatment act. If the treatment act is allowed to play out, benefit is demonstrated more often than not. The risk in most of these practices is low. Although there are anecdotal reports of adverse neurological consequences from manipulating the neck, untoward physical consequences are rare.

THE ETHICAL CONUNDRUM

Much that is therapeutic in the practice of medicine as purveyed by my guild relates to the treatment act, not just the modality, and many of our therapeutic modalities barely pass scientific muster. This book takes its place in the scientific tradition that Western medicine holds sacrosanct and that is embodied in the philosophy of Karl Popper: all therapeutic modalities found to be lacking in adequate benefit/risk ratios should be recognized, decried, and discarded. The process may be inefficient and sometimes contentious, but therein lies progress.

Alternative and complementary modalities are widely perceived to work and, indeed, have a life of their own. They survive in the face of science by relying on the idiosyncrasies of their application or preparation. There is no progress, only the self-perpetuation of the treatment acts. "So what?" you say. Who cares if the modalities are fatuous, as long as the treatment act is not harmful and the clinical effect is palliative? I do. I care if fellow citizens are being duped into thinking that they are participating in a therapeutic contract that is more than magical. I care that I am being forced to underwrite such magical therapies. And I care if people are unknowingly being drawn into a therapeutic envelope.

Life has many aspects that are beyond reason. Poets conceptualize "love" better than neurobiologists dissect it. Religion has a place – and for some a healing place. Ethnic identities, cultural norms, and social constructions all have their place in the fabric of our lives. All can provide for beauty, caring, and comfort. All can have excesses and require close scrutiny in this regard. Individuals must choose whether to participate and how to value these options, all in their own fashion. But none of these aspects of life is supported by health insurance. Treatment acts based on modalities whose effectiveness has been scientifically refuted are not treatment acts; they are belief systems. I am aware of no insurance scheme that sets out to indemnify a belief system. Treatment acts based on modalities that have yet to be tested may also be belief systems. Many are indemnified, probably far too many.

Finally, any treatment act that fosters a therapeutic envelope is lacking. For me, such treatments are anathema. This book presents a strong argument against medicalization. The proper role for medicine is to collaborate with patients in the goal that they will become persons again. If there is no modality up to that task, then the treatment act must compensate. No one should ever be a "diabetic" when he can be a person coping with diabetes. No one should be a "rheumatoid" when she can be a person coping with rheumatoid arthritis. No workers should be told that they have spinal disorders when their illness is more a consequence of contextual factors that compromise their ability to cope with one of life's intermittent and remittent bedevilments. If I am able to craft this case against medicalization, why should I condone chiropractorization, herbalization, acupuncturization, or the like?

Epilogue
A Ripe Old Age

"Man has no dominion over the breath of life, neither to retain that flicker of life nor the power to determine the day of death."

Ecclesiastes 8:8

The overarching theme of *The Last Well Person* is authority – the authority of medicine. This authority is not the same as that of your physician. Rather, the authority of which I speak belongs to the institution of medicine, the organizational structure to which your physician must conform. To paraphrase Robespierre, institutions are born to die; it is the people who are born to live. The twentieth century has witnessed the birth of two institutions of medicine: the first elevated medicine to be the arbiter of normalcy; the second superimposed the trappings of enterprise and created the "health-care delivery system."

Some personal attributes can be considered unusual, aberrant, or deviant, depending on whether they are framed in the context of moral transgression or in the context of disease. If the former holds sway, the attribute is secularized; if the latter, it is medicalized. Suicide and particular sexual proclivities have spent generations in one or the other of these arenas. Alcoholism once was secularized. Today alcoholism is medicalized, by both medical and legal decree; obesity has been medicalized by medical decree, with some wobbling in the conviction. As we saw in Part Two, aging, woefulness, and job dissatisfaction have been medicalized, as has inattentiveness in children. The

medicalization of personal traits is not new; it can be traced
back for centuries. In the twentieth century, the institution of
medicine was called on to serve this function as an agent of the
state. In this fashion, physicians have assumed responsibility
for medicalizing violence, work absenteeism, and long-term
disability.

By mid-century, the institution of medicine had gained professional dominance in the halls of policy and had taken on a
mantle of cultural authority. This cultural hegemony recruited
physicians to the role of moral entrepreneurs. Among the moral
entrepreneurs were crusaders for clinical matters viewed as crucial to the health of the public, or to a segment of the public,
even if that view was a construction of illness based solely on
conviction and subject to self-interest. Eventually this hegemony
created the contemporary institution of medicine in the United
States, a "health-care industry" that influences the thinking of
all other resource-advantaged nations.

I choose the term "moral entrepreneur" advisedly. It is the
transfer of considerable wealth between the various stakeholders
that drives health policy. Furthermore, health policy is rife with
the influence of these moral entrepreneurs, whose credentialing
and peer reviewing are far removed from the bedside and for
whom conflict of interest is subsumed by conviction. Shading of
judgment, torturing of data, and zealous marketing are the
results, and they are all documented, chapter by chapter,
through this book. Authority cannot be counted on to demand
that your interest is primary in the delivery of your care by your
physician. Authority cannot be counted on to succour the Last
Well Person. The institution of medicine is ethically bankrupt.

Part of being ill is to feel the need to seek professional care,
to subjugate some degree of autonomy to a degree of trust. That
is true even today when your professional care might be a fleeting moment of consignment to an impersonal station in the
health-care delivery system. But staying well does not require a
lessening of autonomy. On the contrary, it requires the utmost
vigilance with regard to the conflicts of interest of the moral
entrepreneurs who establish the standard of care your physician

is expected to adhere to. *The Last Well Person* is a primer. The analyses in the chapters will require constant update and revision, and there are topics yet to be probed.

For those of you who aspire to a ripe old age, I place the responsibility directly on you. I ask you never to let your guard down or to relinquish your autonomy when you deal with the health-care delivery system. *The Last Well Person* is, in essence, a treatise on medicalization and what I call "Type II Medical Malpractice" – the act of doing something to you very well that you did not need in the first place. Recognizing the power of these medical phenomena in the current system is a prerequisite to refashioning it to your benefit and to negotiating your own medical care. It is unconscionable that the system has evolved in a way that challenges your discernment. The system must be changed, but the stakes are high and many of the stakeholders are opposed to changes that do not benefit themselves.

As for the octogenarians, to be well at your ripe old age means you have managed to cope with a variety of life challenges. I have written this book to offer guideposts to the generations behind you who aspire to be, like you, well octogenarians. The premise of Part One was that the longevity of our species is limited very close to the age of eighty-five. If you are a well octogenarian, your days are numbered. However, the exact number of your days is not known, just their probability. You cannot know when you will die or what the ending will be. If you are truly fortunate, you will never know either one. You are already a ripe old age. Can these remaining years be an enjoyable and joyful time of life?

Much of what will happen is out of your hands, but not all. Family and community are the precious underpinnings for a joyful ninth decade. This insight pertains to the last decade of life, whether it's the sixth decade in a resource-constrained culture such as India or the ninth decade in the advantaged West. However, octogenarians in the advantaged West have another challenge that relates to the entitlement of senior citizens to the "best" health care money can buy. Senior citizens are a powerful lobby in that regard. Yet, in contemporary society, they are marching arm in arm with the moral entrepreneurs of the pharmaceutical industry, the hospital industry, and the other components of the medical industry. Analysis of Medicare data documents that excess spending and excessive care transfer considerable wealth but do nothing for the well-being or satisfaction of the elderly. All they gain are the hazards of over-medicalization, or iatrogenicity.

My advice to the elderly is simple: Beware of medical schemes that are offered to prolong your life. The only reason for medical intervention should be an acute medical problem or emergency. For octogenarians, the four goals of self-actualization, independence, interaction, and comfort are primary and should form the basis of every medical decision. Beware, too, of the use of pharmaceuticals to serve these goals. The drugs that are available are limited in number and in effectiveness. Their therapeutic indices – the tightness of their benefit/risk ratios – are inversely related to your age, so side effects are almost as likely as benefits. Don't take any drug for these goals that is not clearly moving you in the right direction. Negotiate with your doctor for trial periods that have a fixed end-point. If you are not clearly better by that time, you should stop the drug. Otherwise, you will join the majority in your pill-taking cohort: 40 per cent of the elderly consume five or more different prescription drugs each week, and one out of every eight pill-takers suffers a serious side effect each year.

Standing up to the moral entrepreneurs and the health-care delivery system they have nurtured is a lonely and demanding task. It is painfully so for your physician, if she is so inclined, and very time consuming. Common practices, algorithms (therapeutic road maps), guidelines, and reimbursement schemes all stand in the way of independent thinking. Your physician can arrange for a cardiac catheterization far more readily than he can manage the considerable time to discuss why it may not be necessary. There are many physicians, including my own students, who would gladly assume that latter role if the health-care delivery system made it feasible. If you find such a stalwart iconoclast in the current climate, you are fortunate.

More likely, you will have to take the responsibility for asking the questions about risks and benefits. You will have to demand detailed responses before you acquiesce to any medical procedures and before you believe any of the advice in the media, including the direct-to-consumer advertising of the pharmaceutical companies. It's a lonely task, but I wish you the conviction to take it on and to see it through. I wish you well.

Annotated Readings

PROLOGUE

Karl Popper described truth as tentative at best, the hypothesis yet to be disproved. See his *Conjectures and Refutations* (2000), first published in 1963. David Miller, *Popper Selections* (1985), introduces Popper's social philosophy as well as his philosophy of science. The biography by Malachi Hacohen, *Karl Popper: The Formative Years* (2000), is also engaging and informative.

Popper's refutationist treatment of truth was as discomforting as it was revolutionary. Is there no way to generate more certainty? Epistemology since Hume has sought reasonable compromises that might offer some hope of a valid approximate. Inferential reasoning relies on documenting the consistency of observations, the strength and specificity of associations, and the coherence of theories in generating causal inferences. Inferential reasoning provides most of the "evidence" on which we can reason decisions in medicine and beyond. *The Last Well Person* adheres far more to refutationist principles in explaining how to recognize, quantify, and cope with uncertainty. I will demonstrate, repeatedly, how inferential reasoning has led us astray. I recommend Rothman's elegant and accessible collection of essays, *Causal Inference* (1988), to the interested reader.

Popper's constructions fell into disfavour late in his career, partly because his social philosophy was deemed less politically correct in the post-war era than during the Second World War, when it was written in an attempt to grasp the rise of fascism. His refutationist philosophy of science had to be modified in light of Thomas Kuhn, *The Structure of Scientific Revolutions* (1970). Kuhn explained how a "paradigm shift" caused important hypotheses to be rejected.

The image I use in my teaching is that amid the vast swamp of ignorance are discrete islands composed of rejected hypotheses. At the high point of each island, scientists are feverishly testing those hypotheses that have yet to be rejected. Each island is isolated from the others not just by the teeming swamp waters but because the language and perspective of those labouring on it are unique, constructed around the preconceptions and the histories of the clustered scientists. The scope of the enterprise on each island is determined by society, which looks down on this swamp with proprietary zeal. The hypotheses deemed particularly relevant are socially constructed. When society is convinced that one socially constructed enterprise is more "relevant" or "important," resources are deposited on the shore and scientists migrate there, adding energy to the testing of the paradigm. My philosophy, so stated, countenances Popper's *Conjectures and Refutations*, Kuhn's paradigm shifts, and the social construction of "science."

The "illness of work incapacity" is one focus of my scholarship. See the third edition of my monograph *Occupational Musculoskeletal Disorders* (2004), which dissects the social components of musculoskeletal morbidity.

Medicalization is a concept promulgated mainly by medical anthropologists in the second half of the twentieth century. Kaja Finkler, *Experiencing the New Genetics* (2000, p. 176), defines it as follows: "Medicalization restructures reality by intruding on the world people take for granted, on their tacit understanding of what is normal, by transforming the taken-for-granted state into an abnormal, disconcerting state, separating the individual from the larger whole." She explains how the genomic revolution is medicalizing the concepts of family and kinship, in the same way that homosexuality, menopause, puberty, orgasm, and the many examples I analyze in Part Two were medicalized previously. The dialectic by which the saving grace of genomics has become a social construction is as pressing as it is scientifically flawed. See Hadler and Evans, "The Kin in the Gene" (2001).

PART ONE: THE METHUSELAH COMPLEX

For recent literature on social epidemiology, see Wilkinson, *Unhealthy Societies* (1996), for the concept of income gap; Berkman and Kawachi, eds, *Social Epidemiology* (2000), and Kawachi and Berkman, *Neighbourhoods and Health* (2003), for a general overview; and Hertzman, "Health and Human Society" (2001), for a brief but eloquent survey. Lantz and colleagues, "Socioeconomic Factors, Health Behaviors, and Mortality," support my assertions that only 25 per cent of the hazard to longevity resides in the proximate causes of death.

Some of my own articles provide an overview of the concept that proximate causes pale next to SES and job satisfaction in determining our mortal fate: "Laboring for Longevity" (1999) and "Rheumatology and the Health of the Workforce" (2001). Fitzpatrick, "Social Status and Mortality" (2001), offers yet another perspective along the same lines. I examine this topic in some depth in chapter 9.

The divide between the students of life-course and proximate-cause epidemiology is nowhere more striking than in Britain, and British scholars have set the pace in both arenas. Professors M. Marmot of University College, London, and R. Wilkinson of the University of Sussex are pioneers in the former; Professors W.R.S. Doll, R. Peto, and R. Turner of Oxford in the latter. It is rare for the perspectives and analytic techniques of these two groups to converge on the same cohorts, either in the United Kingdom or elsewhere. When there is convergence, it is telling. Herman A. Tyroler at the University of North Carolina has been one of the American pioneers in the study of the proximate-cause epidemiology of coronary artery disease, probing the influence of hypertension, hypercholesterolemia, and the like for decades. Spearheaded by Tyroler in the late 1980s, the Atherosclerosis Risk in Communities Study cohort was established by sampling adults from the populations of Forsyth County, NC, Jackson, Miss., suburbs of Minneapolis, and Washington County, Md. The cohort was forty-five to sixty-four years of age at inception. During almost a decade of observation, 615 coronary events occurred in 13,000 participants. The poorest whites were three times more likely to be afflicted than the wealthiest whites; for blacks, the hazard ratio was 2:5. These ratios were unaffected after statistically adjusting for established biological risk factors.

Most daunting is the observation that the hazard associates with the SES characteristics of the neighbourhood more strongly than with that of the individual. If you are living your life in a disadvantaged neighbourhood, you are marked – regardless of whether your own income or educational achievements outstrip your neighbours'. See Diez Roux and colleagues, "Neighborhood of Residence and Incidence of Coronary Heart Disease" (2001). We can only guess, at this point, what elements of life in a dismal neighbourhood place such burdens on the biology of the residents. I, for one, would call for improving the quality of neighbourhood life rather than expending energy in dissecting its mortal mediators.

I return repeatedly to issues that relate to evidence-based medicine in the context of each of the chapters. Kaptchuk, "Effect of Interpretive Bias on Research Evidence" (2003), discusses the biases that lead physicians to conclusions that far outstrip those supportable by available evidence. The same biases infect medical journalism, marketing, and common sense – and lead to medicalization.

The Virchow quotation is from Ackerknecht, *Rudolf Virchow* (1953), 127.

CHAPTER ONE: INTERVENTIONAL CARDIOLOGY
AND KINDRED DELUSIONS

A voluminous literature supports nearly all the points I have made in this chapter. The decline in cardiovascular disease mortality is well documented. A representative group of articles examining the trend before the mid-1980s includes Pell and Fayerweather, "Trends in the Incidence of Myocardial Infarction and in Associated Mortality and Morbidity in a Large Employed Population" (1985); Gomez-Marin and colleagues, "Improvement in the Long-Term Survival among Patients Hospitalized with Acute Myocardial Infarction, 1970–80" (1987); and Goldberg and colleagues, "Recent Changes in Attack and Survival Rates of Acute Myocardial Infarction (1875–1981)" (1986).

Even the vaunted Framingham Study investigators were hard pressed to ascribe the decline in incidence and survival of cardiovascular disease simply to a reduction in risk factors (Sutkowski and colleagues, "Changes in Risk Factors and the Decline in Mortality from Cardiovascular

Disease," 1990). Some researchers have made a case for the role of reduced risk factors in the continuation of the trend into the 1990s (McGovern and colleagues, "Recent Trends in Acute Coronary Heart Disease," 1996), but I question that argument in chapter 2. Any attempt to ascribe this trend to the contemporary practices of cardiology and cardiovascular surgery must contend with the fact that the trend not only predates "advances" but is rejected by science one inference at a time, from the availability of coronary care units to drugs that treat disorders of cardiac rhythm. Yet many still try to take credit for the improvement in survival rates (Rosamond and colleagues, "Trends in the Incidence of Myocardial Infarction and in Mortality due to Coronary Heart Disease, 1987–1994," 1998; and Levy and Thom, "Death Rates from Coronary Disease – Progress and a Puzzling Paradox," 1998).

The improvement cannot be ascribed to the proliferation of unproven and/or improvable invasive procedures from the 1980s to the present. The three classic studies that could not demonstrate any important benefit (except for the 3 per cent with left main disease) led to multiple publications: CASS Principal Investigators, "Myocardial Infarction and Mortality in the Coronary Artery Surgery Study (CASS) Randomized Trial" (1984); Veterans Administration Coronary Artery Bypass Surgery Cooperative Study Group, "Eleven-Year Survival in the Veterans Administration Randomized Trial of Coronary Bypass Surgery for Stable Angina" (1984); Varnauskas, "Twelve-Year Follow-Up of Survival in the Randomized European Coronary Surgery Study" (1988); and many more.

It's important to understand the significance of "secondary analysis" of trial data. When designing a large randomized controlled trial, it is critical to define the outcome to be tested *before* the trial is undertaken. These undertakings recruit patients often by the thousands and make measurements by the hundreds over long periods of time. They generate thousands of data points. If researchers start looking for associations once the data is collected, they will surely find them. For example, let's take one of these large trial data sets and test 100 associations for statistical significance. Perhaps you are curious whether patients with right coronary disease who have high cholesterol do better with CABGs than patients with right coronary disease and normal cholesterol do with medical therapy. Assume you test 100 such reasonable (or even unreasonable) associations for statistical significance. Let's say you are willing to accept that any association is probably meaningful if it is strong enough to happen by chance fewer than 5 times in 100 (5%) (as is conventional in an analysis where the associations to be tested were decided in advance). In the secondary analysis of 100 possible associations, 5 will be found to be statistically significant, but these 5 are likely to be the 5 in 100 that reflect chance alone. This pitfall is minimized if you test for a limited number of associations that you established as "primary hypotheses" up front.

Data torturing of the randomized CABG trials has served the cardiovascular industry well, but patients poorly. When a secondary analysis of the US multi-centre Coronary Artery Surgery Study (CASS) was undertaken, it led to the conclusion that angina patients with plaques in all three major arteries, particularly if their heart muscle was functioning poorly, were a little better off for their CABGs (Passamani and colleagues, "A Randomized Trial of Coronary Artery Bypass Surgery," 1985). This conclusion provides the justification for all multiple bypasses. However, it derives from a secondary analysis of a subjective ("soft") outcome in a trial where the control subjects were not subjected to sham procedures. The claim that CABG surgery palliates angina is based on a nearly perfect example of data torturing.

In addition to my own publications decrying the discordance between the zeal for cardiovascular invasiveness and the science demonstrating any benefit for patients, see Friedman, "Coronary Bypass Graft Surgery" (1990); Schoenbaum, "Toward Fewer Procedures and Better Outcomes" (1993); and Herman, "Reflections on Playing God" (1993).

Cardiovascular disease is the largest source of health-care spending in the United States. Inpatient hospital costs account for the greater part of medical spending, and cardiovascular disease accounts for 15 per cent of those costs (*Mortality Morbidity Weekly Report*, 1994). This revenue stream supports the excesses in health-care costs in the United States, including the $792 more expended per capita on administration there compared to Canada (Woolhandler and colleagues, "Costs of Health Care Administration in the United States and Canada," 2003).

Conflicts of interest abound among many cardiologists and cardiovascular surgeons. Arnold Relman, the former editor of the *New*

England Journal of Medicine, decried the "growing entrepreneurship among clinical investigators" (1989; 320: 933–4). One investigator even wrote "conflict-of interest guidelines" in the same journal for interventional cardiology research (1989; 320: 949–51).

For the rivalry between the CABG and the angioplasty approach and the ineffectiveness of both, see RITA-2 Trial Participants, "Coronary Angioplasty versus Medical Therapy for Angina" (1997). Of 70,000 patients who underwent cardiac catheterization for coronary artery disease at twenty centres in the United Kingdom and Ireland, about 3,000 were considered eligible for enrolment in this trial. The eligibility criteria are difficult to understand, somewhat subjective, and certainly won't generalize. Nonetheless, 1,000 of the eligible were randomized to either angioplasty or medical therapy and followed for three years. During follow-up, 32 angioplasty patients (6.3%) and only 17 medical patients (3.3%) died. That absolute difference was statistically significant, exceeding the 2 per cent clinical credibility level I use. These patients were better off, then, if their coronary arteries were not invaded! There was also no important difference in the incidence of myocardial infarction. There was a trivial difference in whether the medical patients were deemed worthy of a CABG or an angioplasty during follow-up; the authors, and the cardiology world, hold up this difference in order to gloss over the strikingly disappointing result of this study. "Progress" of this sort continues apace, despite a growing awareness that trials with multiple treatments and composite endpoints are fraught with uncertainties that are ripe for abuse by any investigator or sponsor with presuppositions (Freemantle and colleagues, "Composite Outcomes in Randomized Trials," 2003; and Lauer and Topol, "Clinical Trials," 2003). For the pressure to establish angioplasty as the standard of care, see Jacobs, "Primary Angioplasty for Acute Myocardial Infarction" (2003).

On the increasing use of stents, see Mahoney and colleagues, "Cost and Cost-Effectiveness of an Early Invasive vs. Conservative Strategy for the Treatment of Unstable Angina" (2002); and King, "Why Have Stents Replaced Balloons?" (2003).

For panels that torture the inconsistent results of the many trials to generate indications by consensus, see Hemingway and colleagues, "Underuse of Coronary Revascularization Procedures in Patients

Considered Appropriate Candidates" (2001). For post-operative complications, see Hannan and colleagues, "Predictors of Readmission for
Complications of Coronary Artery Bypass Graft Surgery" (2003); and
for the prolonged cognitive deficits from CABGs, see Newman and colleagues, "Longitudinal Assessment of Neurocognitive Function after
Coronary-Artery Bypass Surgery" (2001), and Mark and Newman, "Protecting the Grain in Coronary Artery Bypass Graft Surgery" (2002).

For the conclusions of Cochrane Collaboration working groups that
trials funded by for-profit organizations are more likely to be interpreted as positive than comparable trials funded by not-for-profit organizations, see Als-Nielson and colleagues, "Association of Funding and
Conclusions in Randomized Drug Trials" (2003).

The Whitehall II prospective cohort study was published by Hemingway
and colleagues, "Prognosis of Angina with and without a Diagnosis"
(2003).

CHAPTER TWO: FATS, FADS, AND FATE

The literature I am citing in this chapter is a fraction of the thousands
of relevant articles, but sufficient to challenge the inference that primary prevention of cardiovascular disease is well served by the pharmacological perturbation of blood lipids. The West of Scotland
pravastatin study is published by Shepherd and colleagues, "Prevention
of Coronary Heart Disease with Pravastatin" (1995). The ALLHAT-LLT
(2002) pravastatin trial was published with an accompanying editorial
by a cardiologist who lists affiliations with eight pharmaceutical firms,
including the manufacturer of parvastatin, and who ascribes the lack
of efficacy to "clinical inertia" in response to the uneven compliance
of patients who were to take pravastatin (Pasternak, "The ALLHAT
Lipid Lowering Trial," 2002). The reference that discusses the negative
psychological effects of labelling well people as hypercholesterolemic
is by Brett, "Psychologic Effects of the Diagnosis and Treatment of
Hypercholesterolemia" (1991). The FDA has either withdrawn or
appended a "black-box" warning to the package inserts of 10 per cent
of approved pharmaceuticals (Lasser and colleagues, "Timing of New
Black Box Warnings and Withdrawals," 2002). This result is all the

more remarkable because post-marketing surveillance is not systematic and relies on hit-and-miss reporting.

The cholesterol screening debate was discussed by Frank Davidoff, editor of the *Annals of Internal Medicine*, in an editorial: Davidoff, "Evangelists and Snails Redux" (1996). The American College of Physicians published its "Guidelines for Using Serum Cholesterol, High-Density Lipoprotein Cholesterol, and Triglyceride Levels as Screening Tests for Preventing Coronary Heart Disease in Adults" in the same issue of the *Annals*. Considerable regret has been expressed over the observation that screening guidelines are not effective in persuading people to be screened: Edwards and colleagues, "Effects of Communicating Individual Risks in Screening Programmes" (2003). Perhaps this ineffective translation to patient action results from uncertainties over which guideline to follow, if any.

Caro and colleagues, "The West of Scotland Coronary Prevention Study" (1997), published the pharmaco-economic analysis of pravastatin. Rennie and Luft, "Pharmacoeconomic Analyses" (2000), are as cautionary as I in their appraisal of such pharmaco-economics. Much of the analysis hinges on the validity of the calculation of the "number needed to treat" (NNT) for one year to accomplish something – spare a heart attack, save a life from a heart attack, and so on. It is a tenuous statistic for any particular statin study and, also, across studies: Kumana and colleagues, "Gauging the Impact of Statins Using Number Needed to Treat" (1999).

I have qualms about structured reviews and even greater qualms about meta-analyses. They are statistical exercises, semi-quantitative and quantitative, respectively, that attempt to pool all the data from all trials on a single topic and to derive a unitary inference, in spite of the cacophony of varying methodologies and varying results. These exercises require the authors of the analysis to sit in judgment on the articles as to their quality and to weight them accordingly. That's so subjective an exercise that I am not willing to delegate it when the issue is crucial for my patients. We also know that most negative studies (particularly those sponsored by pharmaceutical companies) are not published, so the meta-analysis of all these marginal articles will also be skewed towards the positive. Finally, published studies that were sponsored or executed by people and business entities with a vested financial interest in the result are more likely to favour the experimental intervention than studies of the same intervention by people and organizations with no vested financial interest. That observation is supported by two Danish scientists in the government-sponsored Cochrane Collaboration (Kjaergard and Als-Nielsen, "Associations between Competing Interests and Authors' Conclusions," 2002), and in articles by Lexchin and colleagues, "Pharmaceutical Industry Sponsorship and Research Outcome and Quality" (2003), and Melander and colleagues, "Evidence B(i)ased Medicine-Selective Reporting from Studies Sponsored by Pharmaceutical Industry" (2003). Most disconcerting is the observation that large trials studying cancer treatments which are presented at national meetings are more likely to be published if the results are positive rather than negative (Krzyzanowska and colleagues, "Factors Associated with Failure to Publish Large Randomized Trials," 2003).

Qualms aside, a meta-analysis of the trials of lipid lowering for primary prevention reaches the same conclusion I presented here (Pignone and colleagues, "Use of Lipid Lowering Drugs for Primary Prevention of Coronary Heart Disease," 2000).

I am not alone in decrying the hype of "relative risk" and "number needed to treat" (NNT). Relative risk is seldom as informative as absolute risk; if your five-year survival is improved from 96 per cent to 98 per cent by some intervention, does the assertion of a 50 per cent reduction in mortality ring as true as a 2 per cent improvement in survival? As for NNT, if the result of the trial is marginal, say a 1 per cent improvement in survival in one year, why should I be offered the supposition that I will save 1 life for every 100 people I treat for a year? A recent review of 359 studies of new treatments published in major medical journals found that the majority expressed and emphasized their results as "relative risk" reduction (Nuovo, "Reporting Number Needed to Treat and Absolute Risk Reduction in Randomized Controlled Trials," 2002). Since the "peer review" mechanism is not up to policing this abuse of statistics, the Last Well Person must do so. It's an issue that I return to repeatedly in the chapters that follow.

The observations of Phillips and colleagues, "Statin-Associated Myopathy with Normal Creatine Kinase Levels" (2002), fuel my concerns about the potential for long-term insidious muscle damage from statin exposure. The authors observed symptoms and demonstrated muscle pathology in patients whose serum CK (creatine kinase) levels were normal. An elevated CK can indicate muscle damage – and it was the hallmark of the catastrophic muscle inflammation that led to the withdrawal of cerivastatin (Farmer, "Learning from the Cerivastatin Experience," 2001). Even without the elevated CK, there is cause for concern (Thompson and colleagues, "Statin-Associated Myopathy," 2003).

The literature on the metabolic syndrome is even more voluminous than that on cholesterol metabolism. It not only subsumes that literature but moves on across many fields of investigative endeavour. It is remarkable how frequently each component of the metabolic syndrome is studied as if the investigators were barely cognizant of the related research. It's as if those who focus on the details of carbohydrate metabolism are uncomfortable collaborating with those who focus on lipid metabolism. However, biochemists and clinical investigators are not alone in suffering intellectual myopia. Epidemiologists do as well. The epidemiologists who focus on proximate-cause epidemiology tend to collaborate with the clinical investigators who study particular proximate causes. In that fashion, we learn of the individual "risk factors." There are numerous studies of the epidemiology of various forms of hypertension, Type 2 diabetes, obesity, and dyslipidemias, for instance – but far fewer of the epidemiology of combinations. The development of the concept of a metabolic syndrome is the response to this lack (Meigs, "The Metabolic Syndrome," 2003).

Proximate-cause epidemiology, which has enjoyed recognition and generous research support, provides the *raison d'être* for much that is lucrative for the contemporary pharmaceutical industry. Perhaps that connection explains why proximate-cause epidemiology has been coddled. However, life-course epidemiology receives little recognition from the proximate-cause epidemiologists in their writings and in the design of their studies. Furthermore, life-course epidemiology deals with the structure of society, and therefore offers the pharmaceutical industry and its collaborators little hope of a profitable intervention. Interestingly, not much has been published in this area. The greatest challenge for the student of this literature is to read the methods and data analyses and to wonder how the inferences would change if the design incorporated measures of SES and the like. Recent studies document an increased prevalence of diabetes or obesity in ethnic minorities (McTigue and colleagues, "The Natural History of the Development of Diabetes in a Cohort of Young US Adults," 2002; Brancati and colleagues, "Incident Type 1 Diabetes Mellitus in African American and White Adults," 2000). If SES has been measured, it can almost always explain associations of this nature (Beckles and Thompson-Reid, "Socioeconomic Status of Women with Diabetes," 2002).

The recently published NCEP criteria for the metabolic syndrome (National Cholesterol Education Program, "Executive Summary of the Third Report on Detection, Evaluation and Treatment of High Blood Cholesterol in Adults," 2001), are flawed beyond the fact that they do not take SES into account. Many of the panel were, or are, consultants to pharmaceutical and biotechnology firms – a legal arrangement and one condoned by their peers (National Institutes of Health, "Third Report of the National Cholesterol Education Program Expert Panel," 2001). My reservations are borne out by the publication that demonstrated that a quarter of Americans qualify for the label "metabolic syndrome," whether they are white or African American females or white males, while only 15 per cent of African American males qualify. Furthermore, the number of Americans sixty to sixty-nine years old who qualify approaches half. Yet reaching eighty years of age is a reality for most of their cohort, particularly the women (Ford and colleagues, "Prevalence of the Metabolic Syndrome among US Adults," 2002). Most of these people with putative metabolic syndrome are normal.

For ethnic and racial labelling, see Kaplan and Bennett, "Use of Race and Ethnicity in Biomedical Publication" (2003); Cooper and colleagues, "Race and Genomics" (2003); and Lavizzo-Mourey and Knickman, "Racial Disparities" (2003).

A recent analysis of the cardiovascular risk from metabolic syndrome in middle-aged Finnish men shows little consistent risk in the 14 per cent who qualify by NCEP criteria, whereas there is a threefold risk for men in the highest quarter by criteria that are more stringent (Lakka and colleagues, "The Metabolic Syndrome," 2002). This syndrome grows out of another U-shaped curve, and we have little justification in establishing cut-offs before the degree of risk starts escalating. It is likely that the various component risk factors exhibit synergy, and that the syndrome is greater than the sum of the parts. For example, obesity is a more powerful risk factor when it is accompanied by insulin resistance – Type 2 diabetes (Reaven, "Importance of Identifying the Overweight Patient," 2003). Therefore, public health policy that focuses exclusively on one feature is myopic. That is evident from the existence of, and machinations of, a National Task Force on the Prevention and Treatment of Obesity, "Weight Cycling" (1994). This body examined the possibility of "yo-yo weight loss" and came up with minimal reassurance that it is not hazardous. Perhaps that is because the actual loss of weight is no more likely to lower all-cause mortality than any attempt, successful or not, to lose weight (Gregg and colleagues, "Relationship of Changes in Physical Activity and Mortality among Older Women," 2003). The metabolic syndrome holds many mysteries, some of which may overlap with those that make SES so crucial.

For an overview of the contemporary conundrum on the diagnosis of Type 2 diabetes, see Barr and colleagues, "Tests of Glycemia for the Diagnosis of Type 2 Diabetes Mellitus" (2002). In practice in the United States, physicians tell patients they have diabetes so frequently that it is estimated that a third of American born in 2000 will be labelled "diabetic" during the course of their lifetime (Narayan and colleagues, "Lifetime Risk for Diabetes Mellitus," 2003). In 1997 the Expert Committee of the Diagnosis and Classification of Diabetes Mellitus of the American Diabetes Association revised the criteria for the diagnosis of Type 2 diabetes. One criterion was a fasting blood glucose of 126 mg/dl or more. The NIH panel that formulated the criteria for the metabolic syndrome established the cut-off at 110 or more. These panels, and others, have access to survey data that looks at the prevalence of the clinical manifestations of Type 2 diabetes as a function of various measures of blood sugar. Most of these surveys rely on surrogate measures that speak to diabetes-specific microvascular damage, such as subtle changes in the eyes (diabetic retinopathy), rather than less-frequent and delayed serious consequences such as blindness, renal failure, heart attacks, or death. An experimental literature explores the molecular mechanisms by which bathing tissue in fluids high in glucose leads to damage (Sheetz and King, "Molecular Understanding of Hyperglycemia's Adverse Effects for Diabetic Complications," 2002). The existence of this literature supports but does not test the hypothesis that controlling blood sugar levels will prevent microcirculatory damage. Surrogate measures are convenient for testing the hypothesis if one assumes that they are important measures of long-term risks.

Surrogate measures, such as blood pressure or serum lipid levels, are frequently employed in intervention studies designed to abrogate biological risk factors for macrovascular and microvascular disease, and the FDA relies heavily on them. Yet surrogate and intermediate endpoints are not reliable in many of these settings (Psaty and colleagues, "Surrogate End Points," 1999; Temple, "Are Surrogate Markers Adequate to Assess Cardiovascular Disease Drugs?" 1999). Surrogate measures are seductive because they tend to be more sensitive to change, both temporally and quantitatively. "Hard outcomes," such as death or stroke, unfold at a pace that demands much more patience and a larger cohort, both of which can tax the resources of any investigative team. Hence, we will always be stuck with surrogate end-points – but they need not fool us.

Among the Pima Indians, a long-studied population with a high incidence of diabetic complications, there is no increase in the prevalence of retinopathy till the fasting blood sugar rises above 125 mg/dl. The general US population starts to climb out of the valley of the U-shaped curve for retinopathy above 110. The relationship between blood sugar and retinopathy is predictable, but not that between blood sugar and other diabetes-associated outcomes. In particular, the risk of macrovascular complications, such as coronary artery or peripheral vascular disease, and blood sugar has less clear cut-offs. Here the relationship is more monotonic (a straight line) than U-shaped, with some risk still apparent in the population with "normal" blood sugar (because Type 2 diabetes is only one of the relevant risk factors in the metabolic syndrome). The expert panels are therefore forced to examine the epidemiology of surrogate outcomes and come to a consensus. The consensus cut-off is seldom age-dependent, even though insulin resistance is a fact of normal aging. Hence, the "epidemic" of Type 2 diabetes may prove to be contrived. It may be little more than a reflection of changing definitions, so more people qualify for the label.

The study of intensive treatment of Type 1 diabetes was published by the DCCT Research Group, "The Effect of Intensive Treatment of

Diabetes" (1993). The classic study contrasting diet, insulin therapy, and a first-generation oral hypoglycemic in the management of Type 2 diabetes was published by the University Group Diabetes Program (UGDP), "A Study of the Effects of Hypoglycemic Agents on Vascular Complications" (1976). In this study, the oral hypoglycemic was associated with more deaths than the alternatives. The vaunted UKPDS Group article, "Intensive Blood-Glucose Control," was published in *Lancet* (1998). Stratton and colleagues, "Association of Glycaemia with Macrovascular and Microvascular Complications of Type 2 Diabetes" (2000), published the secondary analysis observing a relationship between exposure to hyperglycemia and important clinical outcomes.

An elegant demonstration of the J-shaped relationship between blood pressure and mortality was published by Boutitie and colleagues, "J-Shaped Relationship between Blood Pressure and Mortality in Hypertensive Patients" (2002). This relationship should temporize the alarm generated by surveys suggesting an increasing prevalence of hypertension in the past decade (Hajjar and Kotchen, "Trends in Prevalence, Awareness, Treatment and Control of Hypertension," 2003).

The MR FIT trial of step therapy for hypertension was published by the Multiple Risk Factor Intervention Trial Research Group in 1982. For a discussion of the way in which diuretic therapy may have predisposed to sudden death in that trial, and why the risk of sudden death may be outweighed by the benefits of therapy, see Bigger, "Diuretic Therapy" (1994), and Heos and colleagues, "Diuretics" (1995). A recent analysis of the MR FIT cohort after sixteen years of monitoring for cardiovascular and all-cause mortality and morbidity demonstrates that SES overwhelms all the other risk factors that were measured. SES is more powerful than "race" (Davey and colleagues, "Mortality Differences between Black and White Men in the USA," 1998).

The classical trial demonstrating an advantage for the elderly from treating their systolic hypertension is the "SHEP" trial. The most recent analysis of this cohort experience re-emphasizes the effectiveness in terms of a decreased incidence of all kinds of strokes (Perry and colleagues, "Effect of Treating Isolated Systolic Hypertension," 2000).

Stelfax and colleagues, "Conflict of Interest in the Debate over Calcium Channel Antagonists" (1998), discuss the calcium channel blocker stain on medical ethics. The trial by Tuomilehto and colleagues,

"Effects of Calcium-Channel Blockade" (1999), is an example using calcium channel blockers to the advantage of older patients with diabetes and systolic hypertension. Adler and colleagues, "Association of Systolic Blood Pressure with Macrovascular and Microvascular Complications of Type 2 Diabetes" (2000), published the observational data from the UKPDS cohort demonstrating the synergy of hazards when Type 2 diabetic patients are hypertensive. The demonstration that tight blood pressure control benefited the UKPDS diabetic patients was a secondary analysis (UKPDS Group, "Tight Blood Pressure Control," 1998). The demonstration that treating the systolic hypertension of elderly diabetic patients is also effective derives from the SHEP study (Curb and colleagues, "Effect of Diuretic-Based Antihypertensive Treatment on Cardiovascular Disease Risk," 1996). The fact that these elderly diabetic and hypertensive patients are so easily and effectively treated argues that they are different from many in the UKPDS cohort. I suspect that the Type 2 diabetes in the UKPDS cohort is a reflection of the metabolic syndrome, whereas in the elderly the Type 2 diabetes label is a medicalization of the relative insulin resistance of normal aging. I am concerned about the tradeoffs in treating hypertensive-diabetic patients with multiple agents, and less concerned about treating the elderly with isolated systolic hypertension. The regimen is gentle and there is data that it will not compromise the quality of their lives (Applegate and colleagues, "Impact of the Treatment of Isolated Systolic Hypertension on Behavioral Variables," 1994). ALLHAT, an acronym for the Antihypertensive and Lipid-Lowering Treatment to Prevent Heart Attack Trial, is a testimony to the current fashion of naming trials so that their acronyms are pronounceable. The major thrust of the ALLHAT trial was the comparison of anti-hypertensive agents ("Major Outcomes in High-Risk Hypertensive Patients Randomized to Angiotensin-Converting Enzyme Inhibitor or Calcium Channel Blocker vs Diuretic," 2002), and the results demonstrated that an inexpensive off-patent thiazide diuretic outperformed an expensive ACE inhibitor and an expensive calcium channel blocker. A third class of agents, an alpha-blocker, was also studied, but that alternative was eliminated early because of untoward events. This result of the ALLHAT trial is consistent with the literature in general, according to two recent meta-analyses of trials that, in the aggregate, randomized 56,000 people (Law and colleagues, "Value of Low Dose Combination Treatment with Blood Pressure Lowering Drugs," 2003) and 192,478 people (Psaty and colleagues, "Health Outcomes Associated with Various Antihypertensive Therapies," 2003) with hypertension to a large assortment of interventions.

The TONE study renders non-pharmacological options a reasonable alternative in the elderly (Whelton and colleagues, "Sodium Reduction and Weight Loss in the Treatment of Hypertension," 1998). This study is a randomized controlled trial in a targeted population – the elderly – whether they are hefty or not. The PREMIER trial was also randomized, with a similar outcome in a younger cohort (Premier Collaborative Research Group, "Effects of Comprehensive Lifestyle Modification on Blood Pressure Control," 2003). Most of the literature on the effects of lifestyle on longevity is observational. The most influential studies are longitudinal: cohorts are assembled, characterized, and followed over time to see if particular aspects will associate with all-cause and disease-specific mortality rates. This voluminous literature is also varied in quality.

For the Nurses' Health Study results regarding dietary fish and fish oil, see Hu and colleagues, "Fish and Omega-3 Fatty Acid Intake" (2002). This article provides an example of the way in which these investigators mine their data beyond the realm of the credible. They have a parallel male data set, the Health Professionals Follow-Up Study, which began in 1986 by recruiting 51,529 male health professionals aged forty to seventy-five. The following are examples of analyses of these two observational cohort studies that I feel cross the methodological boundary to the fatuous. This observational cohort approach, as is true for case-control cross-sectional designs, is more powerful in refuting associations than in making them. The former is limited by the statistical power of the study design – the ability to claim a negative result is likely to be real rather than to reflect the missing of a positive result (a calculation that is based on the efficiency of the measurement of the health effect and usually defines the size of the study population). Positive results are susceptible to confounding and may reflect unmeasured influences. Nonetheless, these epidemiologists considered their enormous data sets to come up with the following assertions:

- There was no difference in the likelihood of suffering from coronary artery disease between men who claimed one to two servings of fish per week and those claiming five to six. The researchers explained this disappointing negative result as "confounding by unmeasured factors" (Ascherio and colleagues, "Dietary Intake of Marine n-3 Fatty Acids," 1995).
- Coffee consumption was safe in this and other studies (Willett and colleagues, "Coffee Consumption and Coronary Heart Disease," 1996).
- Fibre is good for men's hearts. But this study massages the data to the same extent as the fish study above, to come up with significant reductions in relative risk. Absolute risk reduction is trivial (Rimm and colleagues, "Vegetable, Fruit and Cereal Fiber Intake and Risk of Coronary Heart Disease," 1996).
- Fibre is good for women's hearts (Wolk and colleagues, "Long-Term Intake of Dietary Fiber and Decreased Risk of Coronary Heart Disease," 1999), though the science is as unconvincing as it is in the study on men.
- One egg per day won't hurt you, though many may hurt you if you're a diabetic (Hu and colleagues, "A Prospective Study of Egg Consumption and Risk of Cardiovascular Disease," 1999).
- Men need not feel guilty about eating fatty foods, at least not in terms of their risk of suffering a stroke (He and colleagues, "Dietary Fat Intake and Risk of Stroke," 2003).

Examples of observational cohort studies that demonstrate an inverse relationship between leisure-time physical activity and all-cause and cardiac mortality are the studies by Lakka and colleagues, "Relation of Leisure-Time Physical Activity and Cardiorespiratory Fitness" (1994), and by Anderson and colleagues, "All-Cause Mortality Associated with Physical Activity" (2000).

These studies are representative of all the observational cohort studies seeking risk factors that are under way around the advanced world. Now you understand why the scare of the week is in constant flux. Epidemiology is not able to discern such subtle health effects in observational studies in a reliable and valid fashion. That's why observational studies suggest that antioxidant vitamins are good for your heart, but experimental studies find no benefit (Jha and colleagues, "The Anti-oxidant Vitamins and Cardiovascular Disease," 1995).

In a recent editorial in the *British Medical Journal*, Davey Smith and Ebrahim, "Data Dredging, Bias, or Confounding" (2002), warn that data dredging, bias, and confounding are tarnishing the credibility of modern epidemiology. Data dredging is condemnable; the analysis to be performed must be decided and honed before the study commences. Bias is excusable only if every effort has been made to avoid it. And confounders are, by definition, always lurking. For that reason, only robust results should raise our eyebrows; statistically significant absolute differences under 2 per cent, or even 3 per cent, are best published so that they can be ignored. Trumpeting such results in the scientific literature, let alone the lay press, is unacceptable.

The three randomized controlled trials of lifestyle interventions I discuss are by Appel and colleagues, "A Clinical Trial of the Effects of Dietary Patterns on Blood Pressure" (1997); Tuomilehto and colleagues, "Prevention of Type 2 Diabetes Mellitus by Changes in Life-style" (2001); and the Diabetes Prevention Program Research Group, "Reduction in the Incidence of Type 2 Diabetes with Lifestyle Intervention" (2002). The observational study of survival benefit of adhering to the Mediterranean diet in Greece is by Trichopoulou and colleagues, "Adherence to a Mediterranean Diet" (2003).

CHAPTER THREE: YOU AND YOUR COLON

The Minnesota Colon Cancer Control Study was published in 1993 (Mandel and colleagues, "Reducing Mortality from Colorectal Cancer by Screening for Fecal Occult Blood," 1993), after the cohort had been followed for thirteen years. A second article was published after eighteen years of observation (Mandel and colleagues, "The Effect of Fecal Occult-Blood Screening on the Incidence of Colorectal Cancer," 2000), with the same result. Like all publications in this area, both articles dealt only with reducing disease-specific, not all-cause, mortality. Other articles that examine fecal occult blood testing (FOBT) as the primary screening method include the Cochrane Collaboration (Towler and colleagues, "A Systematic Review of the Effects of Screening for Colorectal Cancer Using the Faecal Occult Blood Test," 1998) and the Canadian Task Force on Preventive Health Care (McLeod and colleagues, "Screening Strategies for Colorectal Cancer," 2001). Again, both articles are too narrowly focused. There's also an entertaining debate on FOBT screening between Jerome B. Simon of Queen's University in Ontario and Robert Fletcher at Harvard (Simon, "Should All People over the Age of 50 Have Regular Fecal Occult Blood Tests?" 1998; Fletcher, "If It Works, Why Not Do It?" 1998). Lieberman and colleagues, "One-Time Screening for Colorectal Cancer with Combined Fecal Occult-Blood Testing and Examination of the Distal Colon" (2001), demonstrate the limited screening efficiency of flexible sigmoidoscopy. The more recent literature has moved the debate to the issue of screening colonoscopy: Imperiale and colleagues, "Results of Screening Colonoscopy among Persons 40 to 49 Years of Age" (2002), demonstrate futility in individuals younger than fifty, while Rex and colleagues, "Colonoscopic Miss Rates of Adenomas Determined by Back-to-Back Colonoscopies" (1997), demonstrate that colonoscopists miss lesions. Lieberman and colleagues, "Use of Colonoscopy to Screen Asymptomatic Adults for Colorectal Cancer" (2000), with an accompanying editorial by Podolsky, "Going the Distance – The Case for True Colorectal-Cancer Screening" (2000), led to the zeal for colonoscopic screening.

For discussions of the risk/benefits of colonoscopic screening, the articles by Ransohoff and Sandler, "Screening for Colorectal Cancer" (2002), and by the US Preventive Services Task Force, "Screening for Colorectal Cancer" (2002); are comprehensive. There are several recent attempts at cost-effectiveness analyses, including Frazier and colleagues, "Cost-Effectiveness of Screening for Colorectal Cancer in the General Population" (2000); Pignone and colleagues, "Cost-Effectiveness Analyses of Colorectal Cancer Screening" (2002); and Sonnenberg, "Cost-Effectiveness of Colonoscopy in Screening for Colorectal Cancer" (2000).

Fletcher, "Screening Sigmoidoscopy – How Often and How Good" (2003), shows how sigmoidoscopy is slowly yielding to colonoscopy, and at a frequency of every three years instead of every five (Schoen and colleagues, "Results of Repeat Sigmoidoscopy 3 Years after a Negative Examination," 2003). No one, except, I hope, the readers of this book, seems ready to ask whether it really matters.

The randomized trial of aspirin to prevent colorectal adenomas was by Sandler and colleagues, "A Randomized Trial of Aspirin to Prevent Colorectal Adenomas in Patients with Previous Colorectal Cancer" (2003), and the accompanying perspective by Imperiale, "Aspirin and the Prevention of Colorectal Cancer" (2003).

CHAPTER FOUR: BREAST CANCER AND
HOW THE WOMEN'S MOVEMENT GOT IT WRONG

For a discussion of medical heuristics, the essay by McDonald ("Medical Heuristics," 1996) is a good start. For Oliver Cope, see his brief commentary on the education of the physician, "Man, Mind & Medicine" (1968). No other surgeon had seen fit to question whether more and more radical surgery served the woman or just her breast cancer.

For Fisher and the National Surgical Adjuvant Breast and Bowel Project, see Fisher and colleagues, "Ten-Year Results of a Randomized Clinical Trial Comparing Radical Mastectomy, Total Mastectomy, and Total Mastectomy Followed by Irradiation" (1985), and Fisher and colleagues, "Twenty-Five-Year Follow-Up" (2002). There were very few relapses after ten years, yet there are very few survivors at twenty-five years. The survival data are presented in table A4.1.

Table A4.1
Women Still at Risk / Surviving Disease Free

Inception Cohort	10 Years (%)	25 Years (%)
1,085 node negative	50/50	12/20
586 node positive	30/30	8/20

Half of the node-negative patients are "cured" of breast cancer, only to live long enough to die of something else. Seventy per cent of the node-positive patients are "cured," likewise to go on to die of something else. If you have enough comorbidity, it will overwhelm breast cancer as a hazard to longevity regardless of the stage of the breast cancer (Satariano and Ragland, "The Effect of Comorbidity on 3-Year Survival of Women with Primary Breast Cancer," 1994). The life-table analysis of Phillips and colleagues, "Putting the Risk of Breast Cancer in Perspective" (1999), places the fearsome malignancy construct into the context of life-course epidemiology.

Fisher and his team followed the mastectomy trial with a trial of lumpectomy versus simple mastectomy. The twenty-year follow-up has been published (Fisher and colleagues, "Twenty-Year Follow-Up of a Randomized Trial Comparing Total Mastectomy, Lumpectomy, and Lumpectomy Plus Irradiation for the Treatment of Breast Cancer," 2002). Fisher's result is similar to the trial in Italy, where Veronesi compared simple mastectomy with removal of the quadrant of the breast with the tumour, followed by radiation therapy (Veronesi and colleagues, "Twenty-Year Follow-Up of a Randomized Study Comparing Breast-Conserving Surgery with Radical Mastectomy for Early Breast Cancer," 2002).

All patients with recurrences, and many with positive margins or nodes, were treated to the heuristic of the day – chemotherapy. The definition of a "positive" axillary node has evolved since the cohorts were assembled some thirty years ago. By the 1990s, pathologists were applying far more sensitive techniques and finding that 10 per cent to 30 per cent of women whose nodes were considered to be negative on the basis of conventional analysis were node positive (Smith, "Approaches to Breast-Cancer Staging," 2000). The Will Rogers Phenomenon (Bialar and Gornik, "Cancer Undefeated," 1997) now applied to staging and its therapeutic implications.

The literature on adjuvant medical interventions is extensive. Among the multiple trials, some are designed to recruit thousands of patients for randomization. Large trials are deemed necessary if there is great variability in the natural history or if a small effect is sought. If there is such variability, however, we need science to teach us how to identify the subsets at most risk and target them in trials. As for the "small but statistically significant" outcome, that's a will-o'-the-wisp, for, inevitably, it will be countered by randomization errors and confounders.

I find the trend to more and more toxic interventions disturbing. Metastatic breast cancer is awful and often lethal. However, it is a chronic disease, waxing and waning over many years. There is room in the natural history to do more important harm than important good. Furthermore, the heuristic of "killing" the cancer with drugs appears as flawed as the notion of "cutting it out." These malignant cells can resist the onslaught of chemotherapy so toxic as to be lethal were it not for stem-cell transplants to support the patient (Stadtmauer and colleagues, "Conventional-Dose Chemotherapy Compared with High-Dose Chemotherapy," 2000). Even the standard adjuvant chemotherapy is ineffectual in post-menopausal women, with a modest 10 per cent increase in relapse-free survival at twenty years in pre-menopausal women (Bonadonna and colleagues, "Adjuvant Cyclophosphamide, Methotrexate and Fluorouracil in Node-Positive Breast Cancer," 1995). The therapeutic horizon has moved away from "killing" cancers to rendering their biology less malignant.

The study of the inter-observer reliability of mammography was by Elmore and colleagues, "Variability in Radiologists' Interpretations of Mammograms" (1994), as was the study of false-positive rates (Elmore and colleagues, "Ten-Year Risk of False Positive Screening Mammograms and Clinical Breast Examinations," 1998). The study probing the psychological price paid by these screened women was earlier (Lerman and colleagues, "Psychological and Behavioral Implications of Abnormal Mammograms," 1991). A more recent article (Sharp and colleagues, "Reported Pain following Mammography Screening," 2003) documents the discomfort, even pain, associated with mammography. Thurfjell, "Breast Density and the Risk of Breast Cancer" (2002), provides a brief discussion of the influence of breast density on mammographic accuracy. The article by Boyd and colleagues, "Heritability of Mammographic Density" (2002), demonstrates that breast density is a familial trait.

The literature on ductal carcinoma in situ (DCIS) is somewhat muddled by the preconceptions and beliefs of the various authors. Finding DCIS, resecting DCIS, and irradiating DCIS are enormous industries in the United States. Furthermore, the mandate to have adequate margins leads to offers of mastectomy, with breast reconstruction on cosmetic grounds. The roles of radiotherapy and therapy with the anti-estrogen tamoxifen following excision of DCIS have been elucidated by the recent publication of a multinational randomized control trial (UKCCCR, "Radiotherapy and Tamoxifen in Women with Completely Excised Ductal Carcinoma in Situ," 2003). Radiation will decrease the likelihood of local recurrence; tamoxifen will accomplish nothing. It would be helpful if those who write for the laity would be more objective regarding the science on DCIS. The emotionality of the prose seems to vary according to whether the authors are surgeons, pathologists, or oncologists. See Morrow and Schnitt, "Treatment Selection in Ductal Carcinoma in Situ" (2000); Page and Simpson, "Ductal Carcinoma in Situ,"(1999); Lerner, "Fighting the War on Breast Cancer" (1998); Fonseca and colleagues, "Ductal Carcinoma in Situ of the Breast" (1997); and Page and Jensen, "Ductal Carcinoma in Situ of the Breast" (1996).

The results of Canadian National Breast Screening Study for the stratum that was forty to forty-nine years old at inception of the cohort were published after a mean follow-up of 8.5 years (Miller and colleagues, "Canadian National Breast Screening Study: 1," 1992) and 11–16 years (Miller and colleagues, "The Canadian National Breast Screening Study – 1," 2002). The results for the fifty to fifty-nine stratum were published after 8.3 years (Miller and colleagues, "Canadian National Breast Screening Study: 2," 1992) and 13 years (Miller and colleagues, "Canadian National Breast Screening Study – 2," 2000). No trial of this size and duration can be perfectly executed because there will always be drop-outs, patients who miss screenings, lost data points, and the like. However, the Canadian study is as close to perfect as such a trial can be (Baines, "The Canadian National Breast Screening Study," 1994).

The commentary by Woolf and Lawrence, "Preserving Scientific Debate and Patient Choice" (1997), on the politics that swirled around the 1997 NIH "consensus conference," offers more than an insight into the advocacy for screening mammography in the United States; it provides an accessible analysis of the way in which political debate can distort scientific debate. Schwartz and Woloshin, "News Media Coverage of Screening Mammography for Women in Their 40s and Tamoxifen for Primary Prevention of Breast Cancer" (2002), performed the analysis of the response of the news media to the controversy. None of the relevant science escaped the deliberations of the US Preventive Services Task Force (Humphrey and colleagues, "Breast Cancer Screening," 2002), particularly since Woolf was one of the principal participants. Nonetheless, the best the US Preventive Services Task Force, "Screening for Breast Cancer" (2002), could manage was a compromise posture, based on "fair evidence," that recommended mammographic screening "every 1 to 2 years for women aged 40 and older." To conclude that the evidence was "fair" required acceptance of the results of other studies as worthy to temper the inferences derived from the randomized controlled trials.

The Nordic Cochrane review of the literature on screening mammography (Gøtzsche and Olsen, "Is Screening for Breast Cancer with Mammography Justifiable?" 2000; Olsen and Gøtzsche, "Cochrane Review on Screening for Breast Cancer with Mammography," 2001) found, as I do, that the Canadian and Malmö randomized controlled trials are by far the most telling of the available science on methodological grounds. Unlike the US Preventive Services Task Force, the Nordic Cochrane analysis was based only on the Canadian and Malmö trials and concluded that screening mammography offered women of any age little but an increased likelihood of more aggressive treatment.

The randomized controlled trial is the best way we have for testing whether any given exposure (e.g., screening mammography) is not associated with any given health effect (e.g., fewer deaths from breast cancer). If there is an association, we can only hope it is real. If there is no association, we can hope that the study design was powerful enough so that an important association was not missed. I am always sceptical when the trial is designed so that thousands of subjects are randomized and followed for long periods of time. The only justification for such a large trial is that the health effect is so infrequent and/ or variable that a smaller, briefer trial would detect too few outcomes to allow meaningful inferences. However, that does not mean that the differences detected (or not) in the larger, longer trial can be assumed to reflect only the exposure. A small discrepancy in the allocation of subjects – more in one group have metastasizing tumours by happenstance – can fool readers into thinking the exposure was the explanation. That's called randomization error. It can be avoided only if all the important variables can be measured and considered in the allocation or the analysis. In small trials probing a robust health effect, randomization errors from "minor" influences are less important. However, in large trials seeking tiny effects, randomization errors can never be avoided. The very fact that the Canadian and Swedish investigators felt compelled to design trials with tens of thousands of subjects followed for decades says that the health effect they target is too small to measure and too small to be meaningful. I don't think such trials should ever be done. However, that's heresy. Most leading

epidemiologists and statisticians revel in these large randomized controlled trials. They do not think they are inherently flawed, as I do. But
they are aware that they are subject to confounding and to the influence
of variables they did not think to measure, or could not measure, that
can mollify the exposure of one group more than another.

Olli Miettinen has no quarrel with the undertaking of the large and
lengthy randomized controlled trials of screening mammography, nor
does he quarrel with the interpretation of the Nordic Cochrane collaborators who accepted the data analysis offered by the investigators.
What he opposes is their analysis. He makes his point, using the Malmö
study data set, in a series of papers (Miettinen and colleagues, "Does
Mammography Save Lives?" 2002; "Mammographic Screening," 2002).
He reasons that the supposition underlying screening for early disease
detection is that the treatment of disease detected earlier is more likely
to cure the disease than treatment started later in unscreened patients.
Based on that precept, he reanalyzed the Malmö data to compare
deaths in screened and unscreened women over the age of fifty-five by
year since entry to the trial. His conclusion that there is a statistically
significant decrease in deaths in the women who were screened two
decades earlier, compared to the women who were never screened, is
interesting, but not as clinically meaningful to my eye. The Malmö
study recruited 42,000 women between 1976 and 1978, allocating half
to biannual screening and offering screening to the controls after four-
teen years. Over the course of follow-up, sixty-three deaths were
ascribed to breast cancer in the screened group, and sixty-six in the
control. Meittinen's secondary analysis is based on the women who
were fifty-five at inception and were spared comorbidities, so they were
still at risk for a "breast cancer death" twenty years later. If the Canadian
life table (table 4.1, p. 81) generalizes to Sweden, Miettinen's data
would suggest the following scenario.

Let's assume that half the Malmö cohort was fifty-five or older at
inception. Of these, about 4,000 would be alive in the screened
cohort, and 4,000 would be alive in the control cohort twenty years
after inception, all of them seventy-five or older. About 2,000 deaths
will occur in the next ten years in each of the control and the screened
cohorts. However, more of the sixty-six breast cancer deaths that were
the fate of women in the control group would have already occurred,

whereas more of the sixty-three deaths that were to carry away women in the screened group have yet to occur. If I am generous and I grant Miettinen all the assumptions he has taken, I am still left with the impression that this outcome hardly justifies all the screening and all the unnecessary aggressive treatment. There is little debate that mammography offers too little (see Sox, "Screening Mammography for Younger Women," 2002; Goodman, "The Mammography Dilemma," 2002; and Fletcher and Elmore, "Mammographic Screening for Breast Cancer," 2003).

CHAPTER FIVE: PROSTATE ENVY

Eastham and colleagues, "Variation of Serum Prostate-Specific-Antigen Levels" (2003), have evaluated the fluctuations in PSA that contribute to its lack of specificity as a screening tool. As such, PSA is a blunt instrument and very limited.

The Scandinavian randomized controlled trial was published as companion articles in the fall of 2002 (Holmberg and colleagues, "A Randomized Trial Comparing Radical Prostatectomy with Watchful Waiting in Early Prostate Cancer," 2002; Steineck and colleagues, "Quality of Life after Radical Prostatectomy or Watchful Waiting," 2002). The ecological study of the Seattle and Connecticut Medicare cohorts was by Lu-Yao and colleagues, "Natural Experiment Examining Impact of Aggressive Screening and Treatment on Prostate Cancer Mortality" (2002). An editorial by Patrick Walsh accompanied the Scandinavian experiment (Walsh, "Surgery and the Reduction of Mortality from Prostate Cancer," 2002). Walsh, a urologist on the Johns Hopkins faculty, pioneered a "nerve-sparing" prostatectomy that reduced the dismal complication rate of earlier approaches and drove the procedure to the forefront of options. However, the incidence of complications in the Scandinavian study is well within the range of the recent published experience with the "nerve-sparing" approach.

The British survey of the attitudes of men with positive screening tests (Chapple and colleagues, "Why Men with Prostate Cancer Want Wider Access to Prostate Specific Antigen Testing," 2002) and an editorial that accompanied that survey (Thornton and Dixon-Woods, "Prostate Specific Antigen Testing," 2002) called for "stronger and braver governance ... to ensure that responsible decisions about risk management emerge for areas such as screening, which have such potentially enormous individual and societal consequences." This same perspective is argued eloquently in an essay by Ransohoff, Collins, and Fowler, "Why Is Prostate Cancer Screening So Common When the Evidence Is So Uncertain?" (2002).

The recommendations on screening for prostate cancer are varied and discordant (Vastag, "Study Concludes That Moderate PSA Levels Are Unrelated to Prostate Cancer Outcomes," 2002). In 2002 the US Preventive Services Task Force back-pedaled on its 1996 recommendation against screening to waffle, "the net benefit of screening cannot be determined" (Harris and Lohr, Screening for Prostate Cancer," 2002).

The study of finasteride was published by Thompson and colleagues, "The Influence of Finasteride on the Development of Prostate Cancer" (2003), with editorial comments by Scardino, "The Prevention of Prostate Cancer" (2003).

PART TWO: WORRIED SICK

See Gadamer, "The Enigma of Health" (1996). The quotation is from page 107.

CHAPTER SIX:
MUSCULOSKELETAL PREDICAMENTS

The supporting literature in this area is particularly rich, voluminous, and compelling. For the Quebec Task Force on Spinal Disorders, see Spitzer and colleagues, "Scientific Approach to the Assessment and Management of Activity-Related Spinal Disorders" (1987). For the Clinical Practice Guideline, see Bigos and colleagues, "Acute Low Back Problems in Adults" (1994). And for the New Zealand report, see www.rcgp.org.uk.

Today, an academic industry is generating systematic reviews and promulgating evidence-based clinical guidelines. The Cochrane Library (www.updateusa.com/cochrane.htm) is spearheading the international effort to produce and update systematic reviews; nearly fifty collaborative review panels have been recruited to the effort, including a

Back Pain Panel. I applaud the exercise, though it is not without serious drawbacks. The documents that relate to the regional musculoskeletal disorders illustrate both the benefits and the drawbacks of consigning the reading of literature to someone else – in this case, a committee. The reviews are remarkably consistent, though not entirely. But the consistency probably reflects common denominators in the evaluative process that predispose to particular conclusions. First, the approach to measuring the quality of trials is not uniform and, more important, may not be uniformly valid (Berlin and Rennie, "Measuring the Quality of Trials," 1999). For example, there is little evidence that the results of well-done observational studies and randomized controlled trials differ much in measuring treatment effects (Benson and Hartz, "A Comparison of Observational Studies and Randomized Controlled Trials," 2000), yet whenever they do, most quality scales will favour the randomized controlled trial. Some of the scales have subscales – for example, to measure the quality of the randomized controlled trials based on details of their design and data analysis. Second, assumptions about and misinterpretations of the published methodologies can result in invalid scores and invalid weightings. Moreover, value judgments play out in these panels and task forces as to the interpretation of treatment effects or the lack thereof.

As I explained in Part One, for all these reasons I am sceptical of tiny (less than 2%) effects even if they are discerned in elegant randomized controlled trials. Yet tiny effects are the rule in these exercises. If there were major consistent effects, there would be no need for systematic reviews. Statistically significant tiny effects discerned in elegant trials tend to sway the methodologists who populate review panels much more than they sway most of us clinicians, who much prefer maintaining the autonomy of our clinical judgments (Nolan, "Credibility, Cookbook Medicine, and Common Sense," 1994; Sox, "Practice Guidelines," 1994). Finally, guidelines are more effective in informing us about the existence of debate than in swaying the preferences of patients (Hlatky, "Patient Preferences and Clinical Guidelines," 1995; Katz, "Patient Preferences and Health Disparities," 2001).

There is little evidence that we can do anything to prevent our next regional backache or predicament of neck pain (Linton and van Tulder, "Preventive Interventions for Back and Neck Pain Problems,"

2001). However, there is a wealth of evidence that psychosocial factors confound our ability to cope with the predicament (Hoogendoorn and colleagues, "Systematic Review of Psychosocial Factors at Work and Private Life," 2000; Linton, "A Review of Psychological Rick Factors in Back and Neck Pain," 2000) or to heal, should we choose to be a patient (Pincus and colleagues, "A Systematic Review of Psychological Factors as Predictors of Chronicity/Disability in Prospective Cohorts of Low Back Pain," 2002). This approach has long been my teaching (Hadler, "The Injured Worker and the Internist," 1994), and it is now that of others (Main and Williams, "Musculoskeletal Pain," 2002). Psychosocial confounders are also the reason people with the predicaments of regional musculoskeletal disorders of the shoulder (Babcock and colleagues, "Chronic Shoulder Pain in the Community," 2002), knee (Hadler, "Knee Pain Is the Malady," 1992; Brandt and colleagues, "A Comparison of Lower Extremity Muscle Strength, Obesity, and Depression Scores in Elderly Subjects with Knee Pain," 2000), and elsewhere (Hadler, "The Semiotics of 'Upper Limb Musculoskeletal Disorders in Workers,'" 2003) seek assistance with their predicaments. Anyone who tells you they can figure out what it is that is causing your next regional backache suffers from hubris that outstrips all the science (Hadler, "MRI for Regional Back Pain," 2003).

There are many systematic reviews of interventions for regional musculoskeletal disorders. The article by Hoving and colleagues, "A Critical Appraisal of Review Articles on the Effectiveness of Conservative Treatment for Neck Pain" (2001), documents the lack of informative studies for the conservative treatment of regional neck pain. But there is no dearth of informative studies for the treatment of backache and no shortage of systematic reviews. Some reviews attempt to encompass the entire menu of interventions (Van Tulder and colleagues, "Conservative Treatment of Acute and Chronic Low Back Pain," 1997) for acute and chronic regional low-back pain. Others take on particular modalities: injection therapy (Nelemans and colleagues, "Injection Therapy for Subacute and Chronic Benign Low Back Pain," 2001), transcutaneous electrical nerve stimulation (Brosseau and colleagues, "Efficacy of the Transcutaneous Electrical Nerve Stimulation for the Treatment of Chronic Low Back Pain," 2002), specific exercise therapy (Van Tulder and colleagues, "Exercise Therapy for Low Back Pain,"

2000), massage (Furlan and colleagues, "Massage for Low-Back Pain," 2002), and the advice to stay active in spite of the backache (Hagen, "The Cochrane Review of Advice to Stay Active," 2002). There is a systematic review that supports my contention that no newer non-steroidal anti-inflammatory drug is more effective than aspirin for low-back pain (Van Tulder and colleagues, "Nonsteroidal Anti-Inflammatory Drugs for Low Back Pain," 2000), and another that could find no compelling evidence that surgery was helpful for low-back pain (though perhaps for sciatica) (Gibson and colleagues, "The Cochrane Review of Surgery for Lumbar Disc Prolapse and Degenerative Lumbar Spondylosis," 1999).

Although there are precious few systematic reviews of interventions for regional disorders of the knee, there are some recent telling randomized controlled trials. The trial from the Houston Veterans Administration Hospital (Moseley and colleagues, "A Controlled Trial of Arthroscopic Surgery for Osteoarthritis of the Knee," 2002) should dampen anyone's enthusiasm for arthroscopic remediation of knee pain in the setting of osteoarthritis of the knee. And read about the Swedish experience (Roos and colleagues, "Knee Osteoarthritis after Meniscectomy," 1998) if you think that meniscectomy is sensible because it spares the knee from long-term wear. Non-weight-bearing exercising makes far more sense and is supported by both a systematic review (Fransen and colleagues, "Therapeutic Exercise for People with Osteoarthritis of the Hip or Kneee," 2002) and notable randomized controlled trials (Baker and colleagues, "The Efficacy of Home Based Progressive Strength Training in Older Adults with Knee Osteoarthritis," 2001). Certainly this makes more sense than contributing to the dismal track record of the surgeons. They seem to carry on in spite of the fact that their traditional and reflexive physical exam is invalid (Scholten and colleagues, "The Accuracy of Physical Diagnostic Tests for Assessing Meniscal Lesions of the Knee," 2001), and that radiological features poorly predict clinical outcomes in knee osteoarthritis (Bruyere and colleagues, "Radiologic Features Poorly Predict Clinical Outcomes in Knee Osteoarthritis," 2002).

The literature for the regional musculoskeletal disorders other than those above is scant. One trial that compared corticosteroid injection of the lateral elbow for lateral elbow pain ("tennis elbow" or "lateral epicondylitis") with physiotherapy or "wait-and-see" therapy found that the natural history was the better option (Smidt and colleagues, "Corticosteroid Injections, Physiotherapy or Wait-and-See Policy," 2002). But little else is worthy of mention, and much else is awaited with great anticipation.

For a discussion of the reason for scepticism regarding the neutriceuticals, chondroitin and glucosamine, see the editorial by Felson and McAlindon, "Glucosamine and Chondroitin for Osteoarthritis" (2000), and the two recent meta-analyses (Leeb and colleagues, "A Metaanalysis of Chondroitin Sulfate in the Treatment of Osteoarthritis," 2000, and McAlindon and colleagues, "Glucosamine and Chondroitin for Treatment of Osteoarthritis," 2000). From my perspective, these compounds are a waste of money. At least copper bracelets can be attractive.

For starters regarding the NSAID wars, I would recommend two books for further discussions of, and references for, the history of the development of NSAIDs: Hadler, *Occupational Musculoskeletal Diseases*, 3rd ed. (2004), and Mann and Plummer, *The Aspirin Wars* (1991). The former discusses the FDA and the historiography of anti-inflammatory pharmacology, and it also introduces the COXIB debacle. The latter focuses on the colourful politics of the industry in the twentieth century up till the 1980s.

The CLASS trial (Silverstein and colleagues, "Gastrointestinal Toxicity with Celecosib vs Nonsteroidal Anti-Inflammatory Drugs for Osteoarthritis and Rheumatoid Arthritis," 2000) purported to demonstrate that Celebrex was safer than ibuprofen. The VIGOR trial (Bombardier and colleagues, "Comparison of Upper Gastrointestinal Toxicity of Refecexib and Naproxen in Patients with Rheumatoid Arthritis," 2000) purported to demonstrate that Vioxx was safer than naproxen. The former was published, even though Pharmacia (and probably some of the authors) were aware of data that contradicted the published conclusions (Jüni and colleagues, "Are Selective COX 2 Inhibitors Superior to Traditional Non-Steroidal Anti-Inflammatory Drugs?" 2002). The VIGOR trial may have demonstrated some advantage to Vioxx in terms of gastropathy, but may also have demonstrated a hazard in terms of cardiovascular disease (Mukherjee and colleagues, "Risk of Cardiovascular Events Associated with Selective COX-2 Inhibitors," 2001).

Not surprisingly, theoreticians have leaped to explain the putative COXIB-induced thrombophilia (Marcus and colleagues, "COX Inhibitors and Thrombophilia," 2002; Baigent and Patrone, "Selective Cyclooxygenase 2 Inhibitors, Aspirin, and Cardiovascular Disease," 2003) with a zeal that outstrips the certainty regarding the effect. Academic physicians who are highly visible as consultants to the pharmaceutical industry and as industry-sponsored "thought leaders" have also rushed to press (Strand and Hochberg, "The Risk of Cardiovascular Thrombotic Events with Selective Cyclooxygenase-2 Inhibitors," 2002) asserting a favourable risk/benefit ratio for COXIBs, an argument they base on a contrived attempt to assert safety and to downplay cardiovascular toxicity. Other Merck consultants (Ray and colleagues, "COX-2 Selective Non-steroidal Anti-Inflammatory Drugs and Risk of Serious Coronary Heart Disease," 2002) argue that Vioxx is safe at low doses. I am unimpressed by the data that supports either effectiveness or safety. In fact, I am impressed by the data suggesting the COXIBs are not as safe (Laine and colleagues, "Gastrointestinal Health Care Resource Utilization with Chronic Use of COX-2-Specific Inhibitors versus Traditional NSAIDs," 2003) or as cost-effective (Spiegel and colleagues, "The Cost-Effectiveness of Cyclooxygenase-2 Selective Inhibitors in the Management of Chronic Arthritis," 2003) as older, cheaper NSAIDs. My response is to eschew these drugs because they offer my patients nothing new except unknown and undefined long-term toxicities.

They are also unconscionably costly (Marra and colleagues, "The Cost of COX Inhibitors," 2000); a COXIB pill costs over $2 in the United States, compared to pennies for an aspirin. If my patient with a painful regional musculoskeletal disorder can be helped with an analgesic, I try acetaminophen (Brandt and Bradley, "Should the Initial Drug Used to Treat Osteoarthritis Pain Be a Nonsteroidal Anti-inflammatory Drug?" 2001). If that is not effective, I try an over-the-counter NSAID. If that offers little, I explain that pharmaceuticals are not helpful and offer exercises, warm baths, empathy, and time as the alternative. Americans seem wedded to their medicalization, however, and they consume an enormous quantity of over-the-counter and prescription analgesics (Turk, "Clinical Effectiveness and Cost-Effectiveness of Treatments for Patients with Chronic Pain," 2002).

My therapeutic posture is consonant with the recommendations of a European task force (Pendleton and colleagues, "EULAR Recommendations for the Management of Knee Osteoarthritis," 2000). As I discussed in the text, a subcommittee constituted by the American College of Rheumatology recommended COXIBS (American College of Rheumatology Subcommittee on Osteoarthritis Guidelines, "Recommendations for the Medical Management of Osteoarthritis of the Hip and Knee," 2000), as did the International COX-2 Study Group, comprised of multiple consultants to the industry and supported by "unrestricted educational grants from Searle, Pfizer, Merck, and Johnson and Johnson" (Lipsky and colleagues, "Analysis of the Effect of COX-2 Specific Inhibitors and Recommendations for Their Use in Clinical Practice," 2000). The lead author of this article went on to a senior administrative post in charge of extramural research programs for arthritis at the National Institutes of Health.

The issue of conflict of interest has been receiving increasing attention in both the lay and the medical literature. It is not a trivial issue. We are witness to the corruption of clinical investigation. Authors' conclusions are significantly more positive towards the experimental intervention in trials funded by for-profit organizations compared with trials free of such vested interests (Kjaergard and Als-Nielson, "Associations between Competing Interests and Authors' Conclusions," 2002). There are many viable explanations for this bias. One is the tendency of industry-sponsored analyses to choose unfairly matched control groups or to squelch the publication of negative results (Djulbegovic and colleagues, "The Uncertainty Principle and Industry-Sponsored Research," 2000). The CLASS trial saga is an example of a form of data massaging harkening to our discussions in chapters 1 and 2 of this book. Large multi-centre trials rely on the "coordinating centre" for organization, data collection, and analysis – a position often filled by a CRO with issues of vested interest inherent in its contractual arrangement with the pharmaceutical firm. It is only human nature for a decision-maker in a contracting company to look more favourably next time on a petition from a CRO that generated a positive result in the previous round. Since nearly all these trials are seeking small effects at most, inaccurate data, slight biases, and nuances in analyses are critical. There are well-documented instances of abuses in all such areas.

At the same time, there is little call for reforms to cleanse the drug-testing process, such as the one I offered in this chapter and which is formulated in a long-ignored article (Hadler and Gillings, "On the Design of the Phase III Drug Trial," 1983). Rather, much chest pounding takes place to identify and label potential conflicts of interest in publications and educational exercises, so that the readers, students, and consumers are forewarned. There is considerable concern regarding the perturbation of the treatment act by the trial, regardless of the setting, and the ethics of pharmaceutical marketing. In the same vein, attempts are made to define the appropriateness of relationships between academicians, their institutions, and the pharmaceutical industry. Some of this chest pounding is so illustrative as to be worth our attention.

The editors of medical journals have been debating how to handle the financial associations of authors for years. The comfortable solution was to ask authors to declare all associations that might have represented a conflict of interest related to the content of the research, and to leave the interpretation to the readership. That was the solution promulgated by Arnold Relman twenty years ago ("Dealing with Conflicts of Interest," 1984), when, as editor of the *New England Journal of Medicine*, he became aware that authors of an article on the effectiveness of TPA (the thrombolytic biotechnology product that did far more for Genentech's stock than for patients with myocardial infarctions) were also monitoring the trial and held stock in Genentech.

Declaration was hardly a solution, however, since it assumed that authors could identify conflicts and that readers could interpret them. There is nothing straightforward about this process. Conflicts of interest are part of life, inside and outside the academy (Korn, "Conflicts of Interest in Biomedical Research," 2000). We all have dual commitments, competing interests, and competing loyalties. Which ones need declaring? How can we know which ones bias our judgment or have biased the judgment of someone else? The challenge is all the more confounded for multi-centre randomized controlled trials, even more so when a "coordinating centre" and a CRO are involved. The response of the leading medical journals was to promulgate and publish, as a consensus document, a detailed guideline for declaring potential conflicts of interest and the role of each author in the conduct of the trial (e.g., *Annual of Internal Medicine* 135 (2001): 453–6).

As a frequent author, I can tell you that this exercise is confusing. For example, if, in a future publication, I reference *The Last Well Person*, am I to declare a conflict of interest because this monograph is a source of income? I have searched my soul and I can identify no personal conflict of interest in writing this book. That disclaimer speaks to a corollary issue, however. There is no original data in this monograph – it is just my interpretations of published data. First Arnold Relman (Relman, "Information for Authors," 1990) and then his successor as editor of the *New England Journal of Medicine*, Jerome Kassirer, declared that, for review articles and editorials, the declaration of a potential conflict of interest was not sufficient. Rather, the "journal expects that authors of such articles will not have any financial interest in a company (or its competitor) that makes the product discussed in the article." Recently, the current editor modified that restriction to "any significant financial interest" (Drazen and Curfman, "Financial Associations of Authors," 2002). Jeffrey Drazen, who had been involved in industry-sponsored drug trials before accepting the editorship, claimed that almost everyone with the appropriate expertise to write such articles was disqualified by this restriction. He even went on to define "significant financial interest" as excluding mutual funds and the like, but not "major research support," and setting an "upper limit on the annual sum that a person may receive before a relationship is automatically considered significant" – currently at $10,000. Relman, speaking from retirement (Relman, "Financial Associations of Authors," 2002), decried the policy change: "Editors are on safer ground," he said, "when they prohibit such conflicts of interest altogether rather than attempt to manage them by establishing flexible guidelines and negotiating with authors."

However, maybe Drazen's bending of the ethic is a reflection of these times. Drazen (Drazen and Curfman, "Financial Associations of Authors," 2002) argues that a zero-tolerance policy "would exclude from the Journal the views of some of our top researchers and would instead favor authors who are not actively working in the field." I would argue that not all "top researchers" are excluded by the zero-tolerance posture, and that the fresh eyes of scientists from other fields can inform us all. But Drazen is correct in saying that many a "leading scientist" would be excluded. The financial arrangements between pharmaceutical firms and the academy have become institutionalized. Many a medical school has been subsumed by an "academic health centre" whose allegiances, alliances, and goals barely encompass the education of the next generation of physicians. Several have developed in-house CROS. Financial arrangements between basic and clinical investigators in academic health centres and private sector pharmaceutical and biotechnology industries are now commonplace. In 2000, one-fourth of the authors of articles presenting original, quantitative studies had specific industry affiliations, and approximately two-thirds of academic institutions hold equity in start-up companies that sponsor research performed at the same institution (Bekelman and colleagues, "Scope and Impact of Financial Conflicts of Interest in Biomedical Research," 2003). The money involved is substantial. The potential for the shading of ethical constraints, if not for abuse and fraud, is real (Angell, "Is Academic Medicine for Sale?" and "The Pharmaceutical Industry," 2000; Bodenheimer, "Uneasy Alliance," 2000). The many legal issues (Kalb and Koehler, "Legal Issues in Scientific Research," 2002) are not well addressed by many of the contractual agreements between the institutions and the industry sponsors (Schulman and colleagues, "A National Survey of Provisions in Clinical Trial Agreements between Medical Schools and Industry Sponsors," 2002).

Is it possible to live up to commitments both as an inventor/entrepreneur and as a clinician/educator simultaneously? Probably not (Kelch, "Maintaining the Public Trust in Clinical Research," 2002; Moses and colleagues, "Collaborating with Industry," 2002). For example, there is concern that the physician who is paid (directly or indirectly) to recruit and enrol patients into a drug trial is too compromised to serve as their treating (advising) physician (Morin and colleagues, "Managing Conflicts of Interest in the Conduct of Clinical Trials," 2002; Miller and colleagues, "Professional Integrity in Clinical Research," 1998).

It has been argued that treating physicians must assist their patients in interpreting the barrage of direct-to-consumer pharmaceutical marketing (Rosenthal and colleagues, "Promotion of Prescription Drugs to Consumers," 2002). Sidney Wolfe, "Direct-to-Consumer Advertising" (2002), has further argued: "The education of patients – or physicians – is too important to be left to the pharmaceutical industry, with its pseudoeducational campaigns designed, first and foremost, to promote drugs." Relman, "Defending Professional Independence" (2003), echoes this plea. However, the campaigns are pervasive, persuasive, and part of the fabric of American medicine. The pharmaceutical industry has spawned subsidiary industries in addition to CROS. Site management organizations (SMOS) are contracted to recruit physicians and physician groups to do the trials. Medical Education and Communication Companies (MECCS) are contracted to put together educational programs for physicians. A contracted company, rather than the pharmaceutical firm, often employs the representatives paid to "detail" physicians. All this contractual delegating adds levels to the vesting of interest (Angell, "The Pharmaceutical Industry – To Whom Is It Accountable," 2000).

The challenge is not just to thwart the pharmaceutical marketing initiative (Relman, "Separating Continuing Medical Education from Pharmaceutical Marketing," 2001) but to undo its impact. There is compelling evidence that the extent of physician-industry interactions (such as gifts, meals, and "continuing education events") directly affects prescribing – right from medical school on (Wazana, "Physicians and the Pharmaceutical Industry," 2000). Furthermore, such interactions strongly and specifically associate with requests by physicians that drugs be added to hospital formularies (Chren and Landefeld, "Physicians' Behaviour and Their Interactions with Drug Companies," 1994). I'm not suggesting malfeasance. If not malfeasance, these behaviours are a reproach to peer review and to the ethical fabric of my profession. Haven't we learned that there is no free lunch (Dana and Loewenstein, "A Social Science Perspective on Gifts to Physicians from Industry," 2003)? Some are calling for the promulgation and enforcement of standards of behaviour for the pharmaceutical industry and the medical profession. I am calling for reform of the way in which new drugs are licensed.

Elsewhere I have reviewed the data that supports my contention that, with the exceptions I list in chapter 6, NSAID gastropathy is much ado about nothing (Hadler, "There's the Forest: The Object Lesson of NSAID Gastropathy," 1990). The data was generated mainly with aspirin and the first-generation NSAIDS. However, no NSAID has been convincingly shown to be safer than aspirin, though there is a suggestion that some are preferable in the high-risk subsets. My approach, however, is to eschew all NSAIDs in that setting.

CHAPTER SEVEN: MEDICALIZATION OF THE "WORRIED WELL"

Stone and colleagues published the study of the "number needed to offend," "What Should We Say to Patients with Symptons Unexplained by Disease?" (2002). Foucault, *Birth of the Clinic*, was first translated into English in 1973. Payer, *Medicine & Culture*, was published in 1988. I use the Kuhnian term "paradigm shift" advisedly with regards to the illness-disease construction. Nearly all of the many "paradigm shifts" turn out to be ephemeral (Atkin, "A Paradigm Shift in the Medical Literature," 2002).

In all advanced countries, and throughout the developing world, there are multiple options and multiple providers to assist with pain (Hadler, *Musculoskeletal Disorders*, 3rd ed., 2004). For the World Health Organization survey, see Gureje and colleagues, "Persistent Pain and Well-Being" (1998). Epidemiology has come slowly to appreciate and explore the issue of persistent widespread pain. Hidden in all these surveys are the people who answer in the affirmative to many questions about such pain (Natvig and colleagues, "Localized Low Back Pain and Low Back Pain as Part of Widespread Musculoskeletal Pain," 2001). These people are more likely to be found in lower socioeconomic strata (Urwin and colleagues, "Estimating the Burden of Musculoskeletal Disorders in the Community," 1998) and more likely to seek medical care frequently (Rekola and colleagues, "Patients with Neck and Shoulder Complaints and Multisite Musculoskeletal Symptoms," 1997). In the Manchester study, investigators are using a stringent definition of chronic widespread pain that requires persistent pain for at least three months in the axial skeleton and in at least two sections of two contralateral limbs. See Hunt and colleagues, "The Prevalence and Associated Features of Chronic Widespread Pain in the Community" (1999).

What is the fate of these people? First, they are no more likely to develop any systemic disease, including any systemic rheumatologic disease, than their age-matched cohort without widespread pain. The prevalence of symptoms in the community is stable, with considerable individual variability (Bergman and colleagues, "Chronic Widespread Pain," 2002). In the Manchester community, the majority seem to improve with time (Macfarlane and colleagues, "The Natural History of Chronic Pain in the Community," 1996). About a third don't improve in spite of whatever benefit this third derive from their propensity to seek medical care, a propensity driven by psychosocial variables as much as the physical perception of pain (Kersh and colleagues, "Psychosocial and Health Status Variables Independently Predict Health Care Seeking in Fibromyalgia," 2001). They are the population that the World Health Organization took note of. A quarter manifest serious anxiety or mood disorder before consultation (Macfarlane and colleagues, "Chronic Widespread Pain in the Community," 1999), a number that qualifies for a primary psychiatric disease label in nearly 17 per cent of those who seek care (Benjamin and colleagues, "The Association between Chronic Widespread Pain and Mental Disorder," 2000).

What is their diagnosis? There is clearly a relationship between medically unexplained somatic symptoms and affective disorders; however, the labelling varies, depending on characteristics of physicians, healthcare systems, and cultures (Simon and colleagues, "An International Study of the Relation between Somatic Symptoms and Depression," 1999). The labelling is also rife with controversy (Sharpe, "The Report of the Chief Medical Officer's CFS/ME Working Group," 2002). I am comfortable with "an overwhelming loss of the sense of well-being," a condition where I see the pain as but one manifestation.

The psychiatric literature struggles with this large group of patients because most have no overt thought disorder (McWhinney and colleagues, "Rethinking Somatization," 1997). "Functional somatic syndromes" is the appellation of leading psychiatrists in the United States in this field (Barsky and Borus, "Functional Somatic Syndromes," 1999), a term meant to capture the heightened awareness and amplification of physical symptoms. "Hypochondriasis" labels a refractory subset who have an unshakable conviction that they harbour a serious disease (Barsky, "The Patient with Hypochondriasis," 2001).

Some rheumatologists insist that the widespread pain is not so widespread but relates to tender points, so they apply the fibromyalgia label. However, tender points require the finger of faith (Croft, "Testing for Tenderness," 2000). They are often present in women who do not suffer, and are not likely to develop, persistent widespread pain

(Forseth and colleagues, "Prognostic Factors for the Development of Fibromyalgia in Women," 1999). In the setting of persistent widespread pain, tender points are related to generalized pain and pain behaviour when studied carefully (Nicassio and colleagues, "The Role of Generalized Pain and Pain Behavior in Tender Point Scores in Fibromyalgia," 2000); they are nothing more than a measure of distress. The label applied to these patients reflects the "chief complaint" that is offered, elicited, or heard, and not a valid categorization (Hadler, *Musculoskeletal Disorders*, 3rd ed., 2004; Sullivan and colleagues, "Latent Class Analysis of Symptoms Associated with Chronic Fatigue Syndrome and Fibromyalgia," 2002).

Much information is available about the plight and fate of these people, but there is no reliable hint or common thread as to a biological cause. For the Finnish twins study, see Mikkelsson and colleagues, "Widespread Pain among 11-Year-Old Finnish Twin Pairs" (2001). Other investigators have sought associations with unusual psychological or physical traumatic events, but the results are inconsistent at best.

Most patients with these labels attribute the onset of their illness to something. In one tertiary care setting (Neerinckx and colleagues, "Attributions in Chronic Fatigue Syndrome and Fibromyalgia Syndrome in Tertiary Care," 2000), the attributions heard most frequently were "chemical imbalance," "virus," "stress," and "emotional confusion." For the Canadian study, see White and colleagues, "Perspectives on Posttraumatic Fibromyalgia" (2000). We do know that patients with this spectrum of illness in tertiary settings who manifest an attributional style have the worse prognosis (Vercoulen and colleagues, "Prognosis in Chronic Fatigue Syndrome," 1996; Wilson and colleagues, "Longitudinal Study of Outcome of Chronic Fatigue Syndrome," 1994). But the prognosis is dismal, even for the others, in that relatively few return to a sense of well-being. Pharmaceutical agents and most rehabilitative schemes are minimally effective, if at all.

Given the tendency of these patients to "catastrophize" (Hassett and colleagues, "The Role of Catastrophizing in the Pain and Depression of Women with Fibromyalgia Syndrome," 2000), psychotherapy aimed improving coping skills has been advocated. There is a suggestion that cognitive behaviour therapy might help, particularly when fatigue is the dominant symptom (Price and Crouper, "Cognitive Behaviour Therapy for Adults with Chronic Fatigue Syndrome," 1998; Whiting and colleagues, "Interventions for the Treatment and Management of Chronic Fatigue Syndrome," 2001). The data are not impressive, which may not bode well for effectiveness outside the research study setting or when persistent widespread pain dominates the illness (Williams and colleagues, "Improving Physical Functional Status in Patients with Fibromyalgia," 2001).

Patients labelled with the functional somatic disorders, particularly those who perceive themselves incapable of working, are characterized by the intensity of their idioms of distress and the dispassionate fashion in which they communicate their narrative of illness (Garro, "Chronic Illness and the Construction of Narratives," 1992). They are the most ill people ever described who are spared any end-organ damage, demonstrable organ dysfunction, or specific biochemical abnormality (Showalter, *Hystories*, 1996). In that regard they are fortunate. But that is not to belittle the pall under which they subsist (Greenhalgh, *Under the Medical Gaze*, 2001). Nor is it to deny the Kafkaesque nature of a disability determination process that must question the veracity of their perception of illness (Hadler, *Musculoskeletal Disorders*, 3rd ed., 2004).

Why do they suffer so? Pain can be unspeakable (Scarry, *The Body in Pain*, 1985). However, those who are burdened with persistent widespread pain feel the need to defend the veracity of their experience (Hadler, "If You Have to Prove You Are Ill, You Can't Get Well," 1996). For a comprehensive treatment of the "mind-body" split, see the monograph by Rey, *The History of Pain* (1995). I am not alone in calling for a revision and modernization of this social construction (Bracken and Thomas, "Time to Move Beyond the Mind-Body Split," 2002). As it stands, the medical management of these patients with inexplicable health problems is difficult (Fischoff and Wessely, "Managing Patients with Inexplicable Health Problems," 2003), often impossible, and rife with the potential for iatrogenesis. It is the medicalization of misery (Hadler, "Fibromyalgia and the Medicalization of Misery," 2003).

CHAPTER EIGHT:
TURNING AGING INTO A DISEASE

For a discussion of geriatric back disease, see my chapter "Back Pain" in the *Oxford Textbook of Geriatric Medicine* (2000). For a discussion of the course and management of the acute compression fracture syndrome, see Joines and Hadler, "Back Pain" (2000). Two recent reviews have explored the prevalence of back symptoms in elders (Edmond and Felson, "Prevalence of Back Symptoms in Elders," 2000; Bressler and colleagues, "The Prevalence of Low Back Pain in the Elderly," 1999). Because of all the randomized controlled trials, there is an extensive literature exploring the incidence and prevalence of compression fractures. The figures I am using are representative (Nevitt, "The Association of Radiographically Detected Vertebral Fractures with Back Pain and Function," 1998; Lindsay, "Risk of New Vertebral Fracture," 2001). About 20 per cent of women over the age of fifty have at least one subtle compression fracture (Jackson and colleagues, "Vertebral Fracture Definition from Population-Based Data," 2000).

Individuals who experience an osteoporotic hip fracture suffer high in-hospital mortality (Goldacre and colleagues, "Mortality after Admission to Hospital with Fractured Neck of Femur," 2002; Roberts and Goldacre, "Time Trends and Demography of Mortality after Fractured Neck of Femur," 2003) and leave the hospital to face a high likelihood of compromised longevity and functionality (Hannan and colleagues, "Mortality and Locomotion 6 Months after Hospitalization for Hip Fracture," 2001; Cree and colleagues, "Mortality and Institutionalization following Hip Fracture," 2000; March and colleagues, "Mortality and Morbidity after Hip Fracture," 2000). Elderly women are aware of this prognosis and feel profoundly threatened by falls and by the likelihood that a hip fracture will signal the end of their independence (Salkeld, "Quality of Life related to Fear of Falling and Hip Fracture," 2000).

In terms of the likelihood of suffering an osteoporotic hip fracture from a fall, both the degree of osteopenia (de Laet and colleagues, "Hip Fracture Prediction in Elderly Men and Women," 1998) and the severity of the fall (Greenspan and colleagues, "Fall Severity and Bone Mineral Density," 1994) are well-documented determinants. For the increase in fall-induced injuries in older adults, see Kannus, "Fall-Induced Injuries and Deaths among Older Adults" (1999). For the side effects from pharmaceuticals which compromise mobility, stability, and alertness, see Leipzig and colleagues, "Drugs and Falls in Older People" (1999). For benefits from exercise and exercise programs, see

Feskanich and colleagues, "Walking and Leisure-Time Activity and Risk of Hip Fracture" (2002), and Rubenstein and colleagues, "Effects of a Group Exercise Program on Strength Mobility and Falls" (2000). On the effectiveness of hip protectors, see Rubenstein, "Hip Protectors" (2000); Parker and colleagues, "Hip Protectors for Preventing Hip Fractures in the Elderly" (1999); and Kannus, "Prevention of Hip Fracture in Elderly People" (2000). For behavioural interventions and modifications of environmental hazards, see Gillespie and colleagues, "Review: Multiple Risk Factor Modification Reduces Falls" (1998).

The controversy about recommending dairy foods for bone health is reviewed by Weinsier and Krumdieck, "Dairy Foods and Bone Health" (2000). For malnourishment among frail individuals most likely to suffer osteoporotic hip fractures, see Hanger and colleagues, "The Prevalence of Malnutrition in Elderly Hip Fracture Patients" (1999); Ensrud and colleagues, "Low Fractional Calcium Absorption Increases the Risk for Hip Fracture in Women with Low Calcium Intake" (2000); and LeBoff and colleagues, "Occult Vitamin D Deficiency in Postmenopausal Women with Acute Hip Fracture" (1999). Randomized controlled trials in the early 1990s suggested that supplementation with vitamin D and calcium demonstrated benefit in terms of hip fracture risk (Chapuy and colleagues, "Vitamin D_3 and Calcium to Prevent Hip Fractures," 1992), not just in improving osteopenia. For a milieu that promotes bone health in the elderly, see Wallace, "Bone Health in Nursing Home Residents" (2000).

Fuller Albright first recognized the association of menopause and osteoporosis and first recommended estrogen therapy for women with pathologic fractures (Albright and colleagues, "Menopausal Osteoporosis," 1941). The observation that HRT had little effect on quality of life, aside from perimenopausal symptoms, was an offshoot of the "HERS" study, a study assessing the effect of HRT on heart disease (Hlatky and colleagues, "Quality-of-Life and Depressive Symptoms in Postmenapausal Women," 2002). The study with the surprising result that women on HRT have more back pain was by Musgrave and colleagues, "Back Problems among Postmenopausal Women Taking Estrogen Replacement Therapy" (2001). The two recent meta-analyses of the health outcomes consequent to HRT were by Nelson and colleagues, "Postmenopausal Hormone Replacement Therapy" (2002), and Humphrey and colleagues, "Postmenopausal Hormone Replacement Therapy" (2002). The Writing Group for the Women's Health Initiative published its results shortly thereafter ("Risks and Benefits of Estrogen Plus Progestin in Healthy Postmenopausal Women," 2002). The discussion by Fletcher and Colditz, "Failure of Estrogen Plus Progestin Therapy for Prevention" (2002), followed (from which I garnered the data in table 8.2), and then the politically correct recommendation of the US Preventive Services Task Force, "Postmenopausal Hormone Replacement Therapy" (2002).

Recent editorializing calls for caution in the use of HRT because the potential harm outweighs the potential benefit, even though neither harm nor benefit is impressive in magnitude (Solomon and Dluhy, "Rethinking Postmenopausal Hormone Therapy," 2003). The Women's Health Initiative data support the assertion that HRT increases BMD and decreases pathological fractures to the same statistically significant but clinically meaningless degree as most other agents on the market for this purpose (Cauley and colleagues, "Effects of Estrogen Plus Progestin on Risk of Fracture and Bone Mineral Density," 2003). Some are belabouring the inconsistencies between trials and cohort studies as to the cardiovascular risks of exposure to HRT, which might be ascribed to limitations in the study methodologies as well as to differences in the pharmacological preparations for HRT.

The consensus seems to be that there must be a better way than traditional HRT (Grodstein and colleagues, "Understanding the Divergent Data on Postmenopausal Hormone Therapy," 2003; Gann and Morrow, "Combined Hormone Therapy and Breast Cancer," 2003). That consensus has gained adherents with the further analysis of the data from the Women's Health Initiative reiterating the stroke risk (Wasertheil-Smoller and colleagues, "Effect of Estrogen Plus Progestin on Stroke in Postmenopausal Women," 2003), suggesting some hazard in terms of cognitive impairment (Rapp and colleagues, "Effect of Estrogen Plus Progestin on Global Cognitive Function," 2003; Shumaker and colleagues, "Estrogen Plus Progestin and the Incidence of Dementia and Mild Cognitive Impairment," 2003), some hazard for ovarian but not uterine cancer (Anderson and colleagues, "Effects of Estrogen Plus Progestin on Gynecologic Cancers," 2003), and the observation that the excess cancers tended to be more advanced (Chlebowski, "Influence of

Estrogen Plus Progestin on Breast Cancer," 2003). Furthermore, there is no protection from coronary heart disease, and perhaps a hazard when HRT is initiated (Manson and colleagues, "Estrogen Plus Progestin and the Risk of Coronary Heart Disease," 2003).

For analysis of the quality of life of the women who participated in the Women's Health Initiative, see Hays and colleagues, "Effects of Estrogen Plus Progestin of Health-Related Quality of Life," 2003). The raloxifene trial is known by its acronym, the MORE trial, for Multiple Outcomes of Raloxifene Evaluation (Ettinger and colleagues, "Reduction of Vertebral Fracture," 1999; Barrett-Connor and colleagues, "Raloxifene and Cardiovascular Events," 2002). Riggs and Hartmann, "Selective Estrogen-Receptor Modulators" (2003), have reviewed the biology and pharmacology of the SERMs.

There is a Cochrane Collaboration systematic review of the effectiveness of etidronate in thwarting osteoporotic vertebral fractures (Cranney and colleagues, "Etidronate for Treating and Preventing Postmenopausal Osteoporosis," 2001). The pivotal risedronate trial was by Harris and colleagues, "Effects of Risedronate Treatment on Vertebral and Nonvertebral Fractures" (1999). In a follow-up industry-supported three-year trial (McClung and colleagues, "Effect of Risedronate on the Risk of Hip Fracture," 2001), the incidence of hip fracture in women who were in their seventies and chosen because they were at high risk for osteoporotic fractures (exceedingly low BMD, often with disordered gait) was reduced from 3.2 per cent to 1.9 per cent by daily dosing with risedronate. In eighty-year-old women, also at high risk, the reduction was from 5.1 per cent to 4.2 per cent. These reductions are neither statistically nor clinically significant.

The alendronate data is pretty much the same. The pivotal trial bore the acronym FIT, for Fracture Intervention Trial, published by Black and colleagues, "Randomised Trial of Effect of Alendronate on Risk of Fracture" (1999), after three years of follow-up, and by Cummings and colleagues, "Effect of Alendronate on Risk of Fracture" (1998), after four. Merck underwrote trials in men with low BMD (Orwoll and colleagues, "Alendronate for the Treatment of Osteoporosis in Men," 2000) and found that alendronate thwarts osteopenia and may even thwart spinal compression fractures. Another Merck-sponsored trial found that if you stop alendronate, as opposed to stopping HRT, the rate of bone loss does not accelerate (Greenspan and colleagues, "Significant Differential Effects of Alendronate, Estrogen, or Combination Therapy on the Rate of Bone Loss," 2002). I am troubled that none of these results makes an important difference for well people or patients with primary osteopenia, or even primary osteoporosis.

For a discussion of the technical shortcomings of DEXA scanning, see Nielsen and colleagues, "Linearity and Accuracy Errors in Bone Densitometry" (1998). For a discussion of the discordance between the hip and spine measurements, see Woodson, "Dual X-Ray Absorptiometry T-Score Concordance and Discordance between the Hip and Spine Measurement Sites" (2000). For a discussion of the push towards densitometry and its shortcomings, see Masud and Francis, "The Increasing Use of Peripheral Bone Densitometry" (2000).

The US Preventive Services Task Force recommendations for screening for osteoporosis, "Screening for Osteoporosis in Postmenopausal Women," were published in 2002. The recommendations were accompanied by an extensive discussion of the literature on which they are based (Nelson and colleagues, "Screening for Postmenopausal Osteoporosis," 2002). A similar literature review (Cummings and colleagues, "Clinical Use of Bone Densitometry," 2002) and complementary recommendations (Bates and colleagues, "Clinical Use of Bone Densitometry," 2002) were published in the *Journal of the American Medical Association* by investigators who had major roles in the alendronate trials. The NIH Consensus Statement, *Osteoporosis Prevention, Diagnosis and Therapy* (2000), did not advocate universal screening, even after the age of sixty-five, and stood by that conclusion in an article published a year later (National Institutes of Health Consensus Development Panel on Osteoporosis Prevention, Diagnosis and Therapy, "Osteoporosis Prevention, Diagnosis and Therapy," 2001). The US Preventive Services Task Force and the Alendronate Investigators concur. The US Agency for Healthcare Research and Quality (AHRQ, *Osteoporosis in Postmenopausal Women*, 2001) shares my perspective on these data – and met severe criticism for its stand.

The most entertaining discussion of social constructions I know is the monograph by Hacking, *The Social Construction of What?* (2000). See Blackmore, *The Mene Machine* (1999), for a discussion of the meme. These treatises will explain my bemusement with the remarkable achievements that produced a bisphosphonate to be administered annually (Reid and colleagues, "Intravenous Zoledronic Acid in Post-menopausal Women with Low Bone Mineral Density," 2002) or a para-thyroid hormone fragment to cure osteopenia (Neer and colleagues, "Effect of Parathyroid Hormone (1–34) on Fractures and Bone Mineral Density," 2001).

CHAPTER NINE: HEALTH HAZARDS IN THE HATEFUL JOB

I cited some of the literature on SES and health in countries that are not resource-constrained in the readings for the introduction to Part One. See also Kawachi and colleagues, *The Society and Population Health Reader*, vol. 1: *Income Inequality and Health* (1999), and Marmot and Wilkinson, eds, *Social Determinants of Health* (1999). For the US National Center for Health Statistics compendium of health data on the influence of socioeconomic status, see Pamuk and colleagues, *Socioeconomic Status and Health Chartbook* (1998). For a discussion of the health consequences of destitution in countries that are resource-constrained, see Dasgupta, *An Inquiry into Well-Being and Destitution* (1993). For a sense of poverty in the urban United States, see Newman, *No Shame in My Game* (1999). The essay by McCally and colleagues, "Poverty and Ill Health" (1998), tackles the issue of the influence of SES on health outcomes from a medical perspective and concludes that there may be a medical solution in increased access. That is not the conclusion of most of the authors I am citing, nor is it mine (Hadler, "Laboring for Longevity," 1999).

The thrust of this chapter parallels that of my career as a clinical investigator for nearly thirty years. See my *Occupational Musculoskeletal Disorders*, 3rd ed. (2004). Much progress has been made since I coined the term "Industrial Rheumatology" in the mid-1970s. The first edition of *Occupational Musculoskeletal Disorders*, published in 1993, was a state-of-the-art exercise, relying on inferential reasoning and a scant science to provide an approach to the complex issues that had evolved to engulf the worker disabled with a regional musculoskeletal disorder. The second edition, in 1999, was a state-of-the-science exercise, picking through a literature that was evolving from the anecdotal to the systematic. The third edition demonstrates that the study of occupational musculoskeletal disorders is now the cutting edge of the revolution in life-course science. I have tried in this chapter to capture some of this excitement.

For workers' compensation and regional musculoskeletal disorders, see my *Occupational Musculoskeletal Disorders*, 3rd ed. (2004), "The 'Ergonomics Injury' as a Social Construction" (2001), and "Rheumatology and the Health of the Workforce" (2001). For the psychosocial context of work, see also Cheng and colleagues, "Association between Psychosocial Work Characteristics and Health Functioning in American Women" (2000), and Johnston and colleagues, "Stressful Psychosocial Work Environment Increases Risk for Back Pain among Retail Material Handlers" (2003).

For the historiography, see Hadler, "Workers' Compensation and Chronic Regional Musculoskeletal Pain" (1998). Erichsen was the surgeon to Queen Victoria and published a collection of essays on "Railway and Other Injuries of the Nervous System" (1866). Keller and Chappel, "The Rise and Fall of Erichsen's Disease (Railway Spine)" (1996), offer a readily available discussion. Mixter and Barr invented the semiotic "ruptured disc" in "Rupture of the Intervertebral Disc" (1934). The Johnstone quotation is in *Occupational Diseases* (1941, p. 381).

Industrial psychology continues to assess adverse psychosocial contexts in the workplace. The pioneering work on job stress and strain is by Karasek and Theorell, *Healthy Work* (1990). "Allostatic load" (Kubzhansky and colleagues, "Socioeconomic Status, Hostility, and Rick Factor Clustering in the Normative Aging Study," 1999) and motivational "flow" (Guastello and colleagues, "Nonlinear Dynamics of Motivational Flow," 1999) attempt to measure the state of feeling comfortable in one's skin. Monotony and isolation seem to be less-adverse circumstances at work than disapproval or lack of a feeling of control.

Epidemiological evidence supports the idea that an adverse psychosocial work context is bad for health. Workers experiencing job insecurity are more likely to recall and record all manner of health complaints (Mohren and colleagues, "Job Insecurity as a Risk Factor for Common Infections and Health Complaints," 2003), including regional musculoskeletal disorders. For the Finnish experience, see Vahtera and colleagues, "Effect of Organizational Downsizing on

Health of Employees" (1997). The Whitehall studies document the influence of an adverse psychosocial work environment on mortality (Bosma and colleagues, "Two Alternative Job Stress Models and Risk of Coronary Heart Disease," 1998), disabling backache (Hemingway and colleagues, "Sickness Absence from Back Pain, Psychosocial Work Characteristics and Employment Grade among Office Workers," 1997), and the malignant influence of downsizing (Ferrie and colleagues, "An Uncertain Future," 1998). Downsizing has a powerful negative effect on self-reported health status (Reissman and colleagues, "Downsizing, Role Demands, and Job Stress," 1999; Borg and colleagues, "Work Environment and Changes in Self-Rated Health," 2000), a measure that rivals SES as a predictor of all-cause mortality.

CHAPTER TEN: WHY ARE ALTERNATIVE AND COMPLEMENTARY THERAPIES THRIVING?

Much has been written on sectarian medicine, now commonly called complementary and alternative medicine. See Gevitz, "Sectarian Medicine" (1987). For a discussion of the history of homeopathy, see Kaufman, "Homeopathy in America" (1988), and Jonas and colleagues, "A Critical Overview of Homeopathy" (2003). Wardwell, "Chiropractors" (1988), discussed the early history of the chiropractic; Meeker and Haldeman, "Chiropractic" (2002), discuss its current status, which they argue is at the crossroads of mainstream and alternative medicine. I am less charitable in my assessment (Hadler, "Chiropractic," 2000). Starr, *The Social Transformation of American Medicine* (1982), describes the politics that led to the absorption of homeopathy into mainstream medicine. The quotation from Oliver Wendell Holmes can be found in his *Medical Essays* (1899). One form of New Age magnet therapy, bipolar permanent magnets, was tested for chronic low-back pain (Collacott and colleagues, "Bipolar Permanent Magnets," 2000) without discernible effect. I find the fact that the trial was undertaken, and published in the *Journal of the American Medical Association*, more telling than the science is illuminating. There is absolutely no physical basis that allows one even to imagine a biological effect.

Baker's treatise "On the Genealogy of Moral Hazard" (1996) was published in the *Texas Law Review*. My discussions are complementary

(Hadler, *Occupational Musculoskeletal Disorders*, 3rd ed., 2004). Carey and colleagues, "The Outcomes and Costs of Care" (1995), published a study comparing costs of treating backache between chiropractors, primary care physicians, and orthopaedists. That study suggested that patients with regional back pain who were attended by chiropractors were more satisfied with their care, even though there was no differential in benefit. The fact that patients with back pain attended by chiropractors are more pleased with the service than patients of other providers has been demonstrated in many other studies, including the UCLA study (Hertzman-Miller and colleagues, "Comparing the Satisfaction of Low Back Pain Patients Randomized to Receive Medical or Chiropractic Care," 2002). This differential is generally ascribed to the fact that chiropractors speak with their patients and explain their therapeutic premises empathetically and definitively. However, they are expounding their belief system as to the cause and cure of back pain, a belief system that is unproved and not readily amenable to testing. For their patients to be satisfied, these explanations must seem sufficient and not beyond reason. For me, since they ignore the psychosocial confounders and focus on sophistical anatomical considerations (subluxations and the like), these empathetic explanations are unconscionable. The patients remain "satisfied" while contending with relentless symptoms. Some call it the placebo effect and defend it as such (Kaptchuk, "The Placebo Effect in Alternative Medicine," 2002), but I am unwilling to condone such a defence.

Coulehan, "The Treatment Act" (1991), discusses the chiropractic treatment act. Several authors speak about therapeutic envelopes, usually under a different rubric, such as "matrix" (Hacking, *The Social Construction of What?* 2000).

Discussions of the pharmacology of herbal remedies are now commonplace in the mainstream medical literature (de Smet, "Herbal Remedies," 2002; Ernst, "Herbal Medicines Put into Context," 2003). So, too, are discussions of the consequences of the absence of standards for purity (Straus, "Herbal Medicines," 2002; Fontanarosa and colleagues, "The Need for Regulation of Dietary Supplements," 2003) and of the decision by Congress to consider these agents foodstuffs and forgo regulations about their safety and effectiveness (Marcus and Grollman, "Botanical Medicines," 2002). Some rely on systematic

reviews and meta-analyses of similar trials to test assertions of effectiveness, assuming some greater truth will emerge. Even with such an exercise, a claim of "no effect" should be read as a claim of no discernible
effect (Alderson and Chalmers, "Survey of Claims of No Effect in
Abstracts of Cochrane Reviews," 2003). When there is no discernible
effect, some call for more studies; see Turner, "Echinacea for the
Common Cold" (2002). In my view, if the study is reasonably designed
and no benefit is discerned, we're not likely to be missing much,
though we may well be missing some toxicity.

The FDA's list of toxicities from dietary supplements can be accessed
on *http://vm.cfsan.fda.gov/~dms/ds-ill.html*. Haller and Benowitz,
"Adverse Cardiovascular and Central Nervous System Events Associated with Dietary Supplements" (2000), discuss ephedra alkaloids and
their toxicities. Ang-Lee and colleagues, "Herbal Medicines and Perioperative Care" (2001), discuss the need for concern about herbal
medicines in the surgical arena. As for the benefit/risk ratio of dietary
supplements, Ernst, "Herbal Medicines Put into Context" (2002), does
it justice. Examples of the science include the articles published by
Barrett and colleagues, "Treatment of the Common Cold with Unrefined Echinacea" (2002); Wilt and colleagues, "Saw Palmetto Extracts
for Treatment of Benign Prostatic Hyperplasia" (1998); and Linde and
Mulrow, "St John's Wort for Depression" (1998). The hepatic toxicity
of Chaso and Onshido was documented by Adachi and colleagues,
"Hepatic Injury in 12 Patients Taking the Herbal Weight Loss Aids"
(2003). The Memorial Sloan-Kettering Cancer Center offers a free
Web site (*www.mskcc.org/aboutherbs*) that reviews the data on the positive
and negative effects of over three hundred herbal preparations – a
reliable resource for any reader who feels the urge to seek benefit from
herbal remedies.

Drazen's lament, "Inappropriate Advertising of Dietary Supplements"
(2003), was published in the *New England Journal of Medicine*. Sidney
Wolfe's Health Research Group in Public Citizen, *www.citizen.org/hrg*,
provides well-referenced discussions of dietary supplement injury and
the excesses of the pharmaceutical industry. A recent British trial suggests that intermittent vitamin D dosing is as effective as any pharmaceutical in preventing vertebral fractures (Trivedi and colleagues, "Effect

of Four Monthly Oral Vitamin D_3 (Cholecalciferol) Supplementation on Fractures and Mortality," 2003). Fairfield and Fletcher, "Vitamins for Chronic Disease Prevention in Adults" (2002), wrote an outstanding review of the scientific literature, exploring the effects of vitamin supplementation on chronic disease prevention. See also the review done by the US Preventive Services Task Force (Morris and Carson, "Routine Vitamin Supplementation to Prevent Cardiovascular Disease," 2003). The task force concluded that there was poor evidence to support the assertion that vitamins A, C, or E or antioxidant combinations reduced the risk for cardiovascular disease or cancer.

There is little suggestion that antioxidants offer any protection against stroke (Ascherio and colleagues, "Relation of Consumption of Vitamin E, Vitamin C, and Carotenoids to Risk for Stroke among Men," 1999), respiratory tract infections (Graat and colleagues, "Effect of Daily Vitamin E and Multivitamin-Mineral Supplementation on Acute Respiratory Tract Infections," 2002), or cardiovascular events (Heart Outcomes Prevention Evaluation Study Investigators, "Vitamin E Supplementation and Cardiovascular Events," 2000). There are suggestions from cohort studies that vitamin E may have a tiny discernible effect on the likelihood of dementia (Engelhart and colleagues, "Dietary Intake of Antioxidants and Risk of Alzheimer Disease," 2002; Morris and colleagues, "Dietary Intake of Antioxidant Nutrients and the Risk of Incident Alzheimer Disease," 2002; Foley and White, "Dietary Intake of Antioxidants and Risk of Alzheimer Disease," 2002).

However, antioxidant supplementation can be harmful. For example, subtle hypervitaminosis A increases fracture risk (Michaëlsson and colleagues, "Serum Retinol Levels and the Risk of Fracture," 2003; Lips, "Hypervitaminosis A and Fractures," 2003). Beta-carotene supplementation is to be avoided in the setting of tobacco abuse; this antioxidant synergizes to increase the likelihood of lung cancer (ATBC Group, "Incidence of Cancer and Mortality," 2003). The Swiss Heart Study (Schnyder and colleagues, "Effect of Homocysteine-Lowering Therapy," 2002) is a randomized controlled trial which suggests that dosing with folic acid and vitamins B_6 and B_{12} reduces complications of angioplasty, perhaps because they reduce homocysteine blood levels. There is a suggestion that patients with Type 2 diabetes will have fewer upper respiratory infections if they consume a daily multivitamin (Barringer and colleagues, "Effect of a Multivitamin and Mineral Supplement," 2003; Fawzi and Stampfer, "A Role for Multivitamins in Infection?" 2003). This study recruited patients from two urban clinics in North Carolina, a state with a well-documented impressive income gap. Perhaps this population suffers from micronutrient deficiency in addition to social deprivation and its handmaiden, the metabolic syndrome.

Randomized controlled trials of vitamins and supplements are proliferating. Phytoestrogens are useless for hot flashes (Tice and colleagues, "Phytoestrogen Supplements for the Treatment of Hot Flashes," 2003); and guggulipids, widely used in Asia to lower cholesterol, don't work (Szapary and colleagues, "Guggulipid for the Treatment of Hypercholesterolemia," 2003).

Wolsko and colleagues, "Patterns and Perceptions of Care for Treatment of Back and Neck Pain" (2003), performed the national telephone survey probing the recourse taken by Americans who recalled back or neck pain in the past year. Table 10.2 is taken from this reference. Druss and colleagues, "Trends in Care by Nonphysician Clinicians" (2003), discuss the implications for patient care of the growing trend to seek assistance from both physician and non-physician providers simultaneously. Astin, "Why Patients Use Alternative Medicine" (1998), published the complementary national survey suggesting that effectiveness relates to the therapeutic envelope, the beliefs shared by the purveyor of the treatment act and the recipient. The chiropractic patient population exhibits more self-reported health problems and "mental health" impairments than the average population (Coulter and colleagues, "Patients Using Chiropractors in North America," 2002), an observation that supports my discussion in chapter 6 and in "Point of View" (2000) on coping with back pain.

The science that has tested the benefits of complementary and alternative modalities is extensive. So much effort has been expended on physical modalities that multiple systematic reviews and meta-analyses are available: acupuncture (Van Tulder, "The Effectiveness of Acupuncture in the Management of Acute and Chronic Low Back Pain,"1999), "distant healing" (Astin and colleagues, "The Efficacy of 'Distant Healing,'" 2000), and spinal manipulation (Bronfort, "Spinal Manipulation," 1999; Koes and colleagues, "Spinal Manipulation for Low Back Pain,"

1996). Several individual trials are worth reading. Our trial of spinal manipulation (Hadler and colleagues, "A Benefit of Spinal Manipulation as Adjunctive Therapy for Acute Low Back Pain," 1987) has been reproduced several times, including by Andersson and colleagues, "A Comparison of Osteopathic Spinal Manipulation with Standard Care for Patients with Low Back Pain" (1999). Homeopathy proved no match for sore muscles (Vickers and colleagues, "Homoeopathy for Delayed Onset Muscle Soreness," 1997), and acupuncture proved no match for neck pain (Irnich and colleagues, "Randomised Trial of Acupuncture Compared with Conventional Massage," 2001). Many of the techniques involved in these modalities are based on physical findings that require some degree of faith on the part of the therapist; inter-observer variability is enormous. That pertains to the "energy field" in therapeutic touch (Rosa and colleagues, "A Close Look at Therapeutic Touch," 1998) and needle placement in acupuncture (Kalauokalani and colleagues, "Acupuncture for Chronic Low Back Pain," 2001), as well as to many of the signs relied upon by chiropractors.

There are those who argue that alternative medicine is scientifically grounded, given that no refutation can be incontrovertible and all refutations have a subjective element (Vandenbroucke and de Craen, "Alternative Medicine," 2001). There are those who argue that a healing ritual can have clinical significance to the extent that it magnifies the placebo effect (Kaptchuk, "The Placebo Effect in Alternative Medicine," 2002). The argument is carried further in that the themes of vitalism and spirituality can be empowering and authenticating (Kaptchuk and Eisenberg, "The Persuasive Appeal of Alternative Medicine," 1998; Sloan and colleagues, "Should Physicians Prescribe Religious Activities?" 2000). This line of argument pales, to me, if empowerment and authentication require living in a contrived therapeutic envelope. That's a sad fate.

EPILOGUE: A RIPE OLD AGE

Star, *The Social Transformation of American Medicine* (1982), documents medicine's evolution towards "cultural authority," and Friedson, *Medical Work in America* (1989), its "professional dominance." See Hadler, "Options in Disability Determination" (2002), for a historiography of disability determination. Lucire's monograph, *Construction RSI* (2003), takes advantage of her background as a forensic psychiatrist and medical anthropologist to offer a telling analysis of the moral entrepreneurship that nurtured epidemics of "repetitive strain injury."

See Cohen, *No Aging in India* (1998). Lawrence Cohen is a medical anthropologist on the faculty of the University of California – Berkeley. In this ethno-gerontology he dissects the semiotics of aging in a culture where the aged are few in number. One Hindi word that translates as "sixtyishness" is used, somewhat derisively, to denote a senior citizen who is stubborn and wilful. For our culture, the comparable term might be "cantankerous," but we would not assume that cantankerousness was age-specific, nor would we consider someone who was sixty as a senior citizen. The Hindi construct of "senility" is telling: it does not connote loss of mental capacity in the elderly but the withdrawal from interactive aspects of life, particularly in the context of family.

For the analysis of regional variations in Medicare spending, health outcomes, and patient satisfaction, see Fisher and colleagues, "The Implications of Regional Variations in Medicare Spending," Parts 1 and 2 (2003).

The Swiss TIME Trial comparing medical and surgical interventions for coronary artery disease in octogenarians showed no difference in either survival or improvements in quality of life after one year. See Pfisterer and colleagues, "Outcome of Elderly Patients with Chronic Symptomatic Coronary Artery Disease with an Invasive vs Optimized Medical Treatment Strategy" (2003). There were some improvements in quality of life early on in the year for the survivors of CABGs, but that's a high price to pay (figuratively and literally). The literature on polypharmacy in octogenarians is rich, though it is not complemented by an analysis documenting the toxicities of this practice. See Gurwitz and colleagues, "Incidence and Preventability of Adverse Drug Events among Older Persons" (2003).

Participation in physically and mentally challenging leisure activities seem to advantage the elderly both in terms of cognitive status (Verghese and colleagues, "Leisure Activities and the Risk of Dementia in the Elderly," 2003) and longevity (Gregg and colleagues, "Relationship of Changes in Physical Activity and Mortality among Older Women," 2003). If nothing else, such participation enriches the quality of life. See Hadler, "A Ripe Old Age" (2003).

Bibliography

JOURNAL ABBREVIATIONS AND TITLES

Am J Clin Nutrition	*American Journal of Clinical Nutrition*
Am J Ind Med	*American Journal of Industrial Medicine*
Am J Med	*American Journal of Medicine*
Am J Public Health	*American Journal of Public Health*
Ann Behav Med	*Annals of Behavioral Medicine*
Ann Intern Med	*Annals of Internal Medicine*
Ann Rheum Dis	*Annals of the Rheumatic Diseases*
Arch Intern Med	*Archives of Internal Medicine*
Arthritis Care Res	*Arthritis Care and Research*
Arthritis Rheum	*Arthritis and Rheumatism*
BMJ	*British Medical Journal*
Br J Sports Med	*British Journal of Sports Medicine*
Brit J Radiology	*The British Journal of Radiology*
Brit J Rheumatol	*British Journal of Rheumatology*
Can J Gastroenterol	*Canadian Journal of Gastroenterology*
Can Med Assoc J	*Canadian Medical Association Journal*
Clin J Pain	*The Clinical Journal of Pain*
Clin Med JRCPL	*Clinical Medicine, the Journal of the Royal College of Physicians (London)*
J Am Geriatr Soc	*Journal of the American Geriatrics Society*
J Bone Miner Res	*Journal of Bone and Mineral Research*
J Clin Densitometry	*Journal of Clinical Densitometry*
J Clin Epidemiol	*Journal of Clinical Epidemiology*
J Fam Pract	*The Journal of Family Practice*

J Gen Intern Med	*Journal of General Internal Medicine*
J Gerontol	*Journal of Gerontology*
J Manipulative Physiol Ther	*Journal of Manipulative and Physiological Therapeutics*
J Natl Cancer Inst	*Journal of the National Cancer Institute*
J Occup Environ Med	*Journal of Occupational and Environmental Medicine*
J Rehabil Med	*Journal of Rehabilitation Medicine*
J Rheumatol	*The Journal of Rheumatology*
JAMA	*The Journal of the American Medical Association*
MMWR	*Morbidity and Mortality Weekly Report*
N Engl J Med	*New England Journal of Medicine*
Neurol Clin	*Neurologic Clinics*
NZ Med J	*New Zealand Medical Journal*
Osteoporos Int	*Osteoporosis International*
Perspectives Biol Med	*Perspectives in Biology and Medicine*
Psychol Med	*Psychological Medicine*
Rheum Dis Clin of North Am	*Rheumatic Diseases Clinics of North America*
Scand J Rheumatol	*Scandinavian Journal of Rheumatology*
Scand J Work Environ Health	*Scandinavian Journal of Work, Environment and Health*
South Med J	*Southern Medical Journal*
Stress Med	*Stress Medicine*

Ackerknecht EH. *Rudolf Virchow.* Madison: University of Wisconsin Press, 1953.

Adachi M, Saito H, Kobayashi H, et al. Hepatic injury in 12 patients taking the herbal weight loss aids chaso or onshido. *Ann Intern Med* 2003; 139: 488–92.

Adler AI, Stratton IM, Andrew H, et al. Association of systolic blood pressure with macrovascular and microvascular complications of type 2 diabetes (UKPDS 36): prospective observational study. *BMJ* 2000; 321: 412–9.

AHRQ. *Osteoporosis in Postmenopausal Women: Diagnosis and Monitoring. Summary.* Evidence Report/Technology Assessment: Number 28: AHRQ Publication 01-E031; February 2001. Rockville, MD. Agency for Healthcare Research and Quality; *www.ahrq.gov/clinic/ osteosum.htm*

Albright F, Smith PH, Richardson AM. Menopausal osteoporosis. *JAMA* 1941; 22: 2465–74.

Alderson P, Chalmers I. Survey of claims of no effect in abstracts of Cochrane reviews. *BMJ* 2003; 326: 475.

ALLHAT. Major outcomes in high-risk hypertensive patients randomized to angiotensin-converting enzyme inhibitor or calcium channel blocker vs diuretic. *JAMA* 2002; 288: 2981–97.

ALLHAT-LLT. Major outcomes in moderately hypercholesterolemic, hypertensive patients randomized to pravastatin vs usual care. *JAMA* 2002; 288: 2998–3007.

Als-Nielsen B, Chen W, Gluud C, Kjaergard LL. Association of funding and conclusions in randomized drug trials. *JAMA* 2003; 290: 921–8.

American College of Rheumatology Subcommittee on Osteoarthritis Guidelines. Recommendations for the medical management of osteoarthritis of the hip and knee: 2000 update. *Arthritis Rheum* 2000; 45: 1905–15.

Andersen LB, Schnohr P, Schroll M, Hein HO. All-cause mortality associated with physical activity during leisure time, work, sports, and cycling to work. *Arch Intern Med* 2000; 160: 1621–8.

Anderson GL, Judd HL, Kaunitz AM, et al. Effects of estrogen plus progestin on gynecologic cancers and associated diagnostic procedures. *JAMA* 2003; 290: 1739–48.

Andersson GBJ, Lucente T, Davis AM, et al. A comparison of osteopathic spinal manipulation with standard care for patients with low back pain. *N Engl J Med* 1999; 341: 1426–31.

Angell M. Is academic medicine for sale? *N Engl J Med* 2000; 342: 1516–8.

Angell M. The pharmaceutical industry – to whom is it accountable? *N Engl J Med* 2000; 342: 1902–4.

Ang-Lee MK, Moss J, Yuan C-S. Herbal medicines and perioperative care. *JAMA* 2001; 286: 208–16.

Appel LJ, Moore TJ, Obarzanek E, et al. A clinical trial of the effects of dietary patterns on blood pressure. *N Engl J Med* 1997; 336: 1117–24.

Applegate WB, Pressel S, Wittes J, et al. Impact of the treatment of isolated systolic hypertension on behavioral variables: results from the Systolic Hypertension in the Elderly Program. *Arch Intern Med* 1994; 154: 2154–60.

Ascherio A, Rimm EB, Hernán MA, et al. Relation of consumption of vitamin E, vitamin C, and carotenoids to risk for stroke among men in the United States. *Ann Intern Med* 1999; 130: 963–70.

Ascherio A, Rimm EB, Stampfer MJ, et al. Dietary intake of marine n-3 fatty acids, fish intake and the risk of coronary artery disease among men. *N Engl J Med* 1995; 332: 977–82.

Assenfeldt WJJ, Morton SC, Yu EI, Suttorp MJ, Shekelle PG. Spinal manipulative therapy for low back pain. *Ann Intern Med* 2003; 138: 871–81.

Astin JA. Why patients use alternative medicine. *JAMA* 1998; 279: 1548–53.

Astin JA, Harkness E, Ernst E. The efficacy of "distant healing": a systematic review of randomized trials. *Ann Intern Med* 2000; 132: 903–10.

ATBC Group. Incidence of cancer and mortality following α-tocopherol and β-carotene supplementation. *JAMA* 2003; 290: 476–85.

Atkin PA. A paradigm shift in the medical literature. *BMJ* 2002; 325: 1450–1.

Babcock LJ, Lewis M, Hay EM, et al. Chronic shoulder pain in the community: a syndrome of disability or distress? *Ann Rheum Dis* 2002; 61: 128–31.

Baigent C, Patrono C. Selective cyclooxygenase 2 inhibitors, aspirin, and cardiovascular disease. *Arthritis Rheum* 2003; 48: 12–20.

Baines CJ. The Canadian National Breast Screening Study: a perspective on criticisms. *Ann Intern Med* 1994; 120: 326–34.

Baker KR, Nelson ME, Felson DT, et al. The efficacy of home based progressive strength training in older adults with knee osteo-arthritis: a randomized controlled trial. *J Rheumatol* 2001; 28: 1655–65.

Baker T. On the genealogy of moral hazard. *Texas Law Review* 1996; 75: 237–92.

Baron JA, Cole BF, Sandler RS, et al. A randomized trial of aspirin to prevent colorectal adenomas. *N Engl J Med* 2003; 348: 891–9.

Barr RG, Nathan DM, Meigs JB, Singer DE. Tests of glycemia for the diagnosis of type 2 diabetes mellitus. *Ann Intern Med* 2002; 137: 263–72.

Barrett BP, Brown RL, Locken K, et al. Treatment of the common cold with unrefined echinacea. *Ann Intern Med* 2002; 137: 939–46.

Barrett-Connor E, Grady D, Sashegyi A, et al. Raloxifene and cardiovascular events in osteoporotic postmenopausal women. *JAMA* 2002; 287: 847–57.

Barringer TA, Kirk JK, Santaniello AC, Foley KL, Michielutte R. Effect of a multivitamin and mineral supplement on infection and quality of life. *Ann Intern Med* 2003; 138: 365–71.

Barsky AJ. The patient with hypochondriasis. *N Engl J Med* 2001; 345: 1395–9.

Barsky AJ, Borus JF. Functional somatic syndromes. *Ann Intern Med* 1999; 130: 910–21.

Bates DW, Black DM, Cummings SR. Clinical use of bone densitometry: clinical applications. *JAMA* 2002; 288: 1898–900.

Beckles GLA, Thompson-Reid PE. Socioeconomic status of women with diabetes – United States, 2000. *MMWR* 2002; 51: 147–59.

Bekelman JE, Li Y, Gross CP. Scope and impact of financial conflicts of interest in biomedical research: a systematic review. *JAMA* 2003; 289: 454–65.

Benjamin S, Morris S, McBeth J, et al. The association between chronic widespread pain and mental disorder. *Arthritis Rheum* 2000; 43: 561–7.

Bergman S, Herrström P, Jacobsson LTH, Petersson IF. Chronic widespread pain: a three year followup of pain distribution and risk factors. *J Rheumatol* 2002; 29: 818–25.

Berkman L, Kawachi I, eds. *Social Epidemiology*. Oxford: Oxford University Press, 2000.

Benson K, Hartz AJ. A comparison of observational studies and randomized controlled trials. *N Engl J Med* 2000; 342: 1878–86.

Berlin JA, Rennie D. Measuring the quality of trials. *JAMA* 1999; 282: 1083–5.

Bialar JC, Gornik HL. Cancer undefeated. *N Engl J Med* 1997; 336: 1569–74.

Bigger JT. Diuretic therapy, hypertension, and cardiac arrest. *N Engl J Med* 1994; 330: 1899–1900.

Bigos SJ, Bowyer OR, Braen GR, et al. *Acute Low Back Problems in Adults*. US Department of Health and Human Services, AHCPR Publ. No. 95-0642, 1994.

Billroth T. *The Medical Sciences in the German Universities: A Study in the History of Civilization.* New York: Macmillan, 1924.

Black DM, Cummings SR, Karpf DB, et al. Randomised trial of effect of alendronate on risk of fracture in women with existing vertebral fractures. *Lancet* 1996; 348: 1535–41.

Blackmore S. *The Meme Machine.* Oxford: Oxford University Press, 1999.

Bodenheimer T. Uneasy alliance: clinical investigators and the pharmaceutical industry. *N Engl J Med* 2000; 342: 1539–43.

Bombardier C, Laine L, Reicin A, et al. Comparison of upper gastrointestinal toxicity of refecoxib and naproxen in patients with rheumatoid arthritis. *N Engl J Med* 2000; 343: 1520–8.

Bonadonna G, Valagussa P, Moliterni A, et al. Adjuvant cyclophosphamide, methotrexate and fluorouracil in node-positive breast cancer. *N Engl J Med* 1995; 332: 901–6.

Borg V, Kristensen TS, Burr H. Work environment and changes in self-rated health: a five year follow-up study. *Stress Med* 2000; 16: 37–47.

Bosma H, Peter R, Siegrist J, Marmot M. Two alternative job stress models and risk of coronary heart disease. *Am J Public Health* 1998; 88: 68–74.

Boutitie F, Gueyffier F, Pocock S, et al. J-shaped relationship between blood pressure and mortality in hypertensive patients: new insights from a meta-analysis of individual-patient data. *Ann Intern Med* 2002; 136: 438–48.

Boyd NF, Dite GS, Stone J, et al. Heritability of mammographic density, a risk factor for breast cancer. *N Engl J Med* 2002; 347: 886–94.

Bracken P, Thomas P. Time to move beyond the mind-body split. *BMJ* 2002; 325: 1433–4.

Brancati FL, Kao WHL, Folsom AR, et al. Incident type 1 diabetes mellitus in African American and white adults. *JAMA* 2000; 283: 2253–9.

Brandt KD, Bradley JD. Should the initial drug used to treat osteoarthritis pain be a nonsteroidal anti-inflammatory drug? *J Rheumatol* 2001; 28: 467–73.

Brandt KD, Heilman DK, Slemenda C, et al. A comparison of lower extremity muscle strength, obesity, and depression scores in elderly subjects with knee pain with and without radiographic evidence of knee osteoarthritis. *J Rheumatol* 2000; 27: 1937–46.

Bressler HB, Keyes WJ, Rochon PA, Badley E. The prevalence of low back pain in the elderly. *Spine* 1999; 24: 1813–9.

Brett AS. Psychologic effects of the diagnosis and treatment of hyper-cholesterolemia: lessons from case studies. *Am J Med* 1991; 91: 642–7.

Bronfort G. Spinal manipulation: current state of research and its indications. *Neurol Clin* 1999; 17: 91–111.

Brosseau L, Milne S, Robinson V, et al. Efficacy of the transcutaneous electrical nerve stimulation for the treatment of chronic low back pain. *Spine* 2002; 27: 596–603.

Bruyere O, Honore A, Rovati LC, et al. Radiologic features poorly predict clinical outcomes in knee osteoarthritis. *Scand J Rheumatol* 2002; 31: 13–6.

Cannon WB. *The Wisdom of the Body.* New York: WW Norton, 1932.

Carey TS, Garrett J, Jackman A, et al. The outcomes and costs of care for acute low back pain among patients seen by primary care practitioners, chiropractors and orthopedic surgeons. *N Engl J Med* 1995; 333: 913–7.

Caro J, Klittich W, McGuire A, et al. The West of Scotland coronary prevention study: economic benefit analysis of primary prevention with pravastatin. *BMJ* 1997; 315: 1577–82.

CASS Principal Investigators. Myocardial infarction and mortality in the coronary artery surgery study (CASS) randomized trial. *N Engl J Med* 1984; 310: 750–8.

Cauley JA, Robbins J, Chen Z, et al. Effects of estrogen plus progestin on risk of fracture and bone mineral density. *JAMA* 2003; 290: 1729–38.

Chapple A, Ziebland S, Shepperd S, et al. Why men with prostate cancer want wider access to prostate specific antigen testing: qualitative study. *BMJ* 2002; 325: 737–9.

Chapuy MC, Arlot ME, Dubœuf F, et al. Vitamin D_3 and calcium to prevent hip fractures in elderly women. *N Engl J Med* 1992; 327: 1637–42.

Cheng Y, Kawachi I, Coakley EH, et al. Association between psycho-social work characteristics and health functioning in American women: prospective study. *BMJ* 2000; 320: 1432–6.

Cherkin DC, Sherman KJ, Deyo RA, Shekelle PG. A review of the evidence for the effectiveness, safety, and cost of acupuncture, massage therapy, and spinal manipulation for back pain. *Ann Intern Med* 2003; 138: 898–906.

Chlebowski RT, Hendrix SL, Langer RD, et al. Influence of estrogen plus progestin on breast cancer and mammography in healthy postmenopausal women. *JAMA* 2003; 290: 3243–53.

Chren M-M, Landefeld S. Physicians' behavior and their interactions with drug companies. *JAMA* 1994; 271: 684–9.

Cohen L. *No Aging in India.* Berkeley: University of California Press, 1998.

Collacott EA, Zimmerman JT, White DW, Rindone JP. Bipolar permanent magnets for the treatment of chronic low back pain. *JAMA* 2000; 283: 1322–5.

Cooper RS, Kaufman JS, Ward R. Race and genomics. *N Engl J Med* 2003; 348: 1166–70.

Cope O. *Man, Mind & Medicine.* Philadelphia: Lippincott, 1968.

Coulehan JL. The treatment act: an analysis of the clinical art in chiropractic. *J Manipulative Physiol Ther* 1991; 14: 5–13.

Coulter ID, Hurwitz EL, Adams AH, et al. Patients using chiropractors in North America. *Spine* 2002; 27: 291–8.

Cranney A, Welch V, Adachi JD, et al. Etidronate for treating and preventing postmenopausal osteoporosis. *Cochrane Database Syst Rev* 2001; (4): CD003376 (25 March 2001).

Cree M, Solkolne CL, Belseck E, et al. Mortality and institutionalization following hip fracture. *J Am Geriatr Soc* 2000; 48: 283–8.

Croft P. Testing for tenderness: what's the point? *J Rheumatol* 2000; 27: 2531–3.

Cummings SR, Bates DB, Black DM. Clinical use of bone densitometry: scientific review. *JAMA* 2002; 288: 1889–97.

Cummings SR, Black DM, Thompson DE, et al. Effect of alendronate on risk of fracture in women with low bone density but without vertebral fractures. *JAMA* 1998; 280: 2077–82.

Curb JD, Pressel SL, Cutler JA, et al. Effect of diuretic-based antihypertensive treatment on cardiovascular disease risk in older diabetic patients with isolated systolic hypertension. *JAMA* 1996; 276: 1886–92.

Dana J, Loewenstein G. A social science perspective on gifts to physicians from industry. *JAMA* 2003; 290: 252–5.

Dasgupta P. *An Inquiry into Well-Being and Destitution*. Oxford: Clarendon Press, 1993.

Davey Smith G, Ebrahim S. Data dredging, bias, or confounding. *BMJ* 2002; 325: 1437–8.

Davey Smith G, Neaton JD, Wentworth D, et al. Mortality differences between black and white men in the USA: contribution of income and other risk factors among men screened for the MRFIT. *Lancet* 1998; 351: 934–9.

Davidoff F. Evangelists and snails redux: the case of cholesterol screening. *Ann Intern Med* 1996; 124: 312–4.

DCCT Research Group. The effect of intensive treatment of diabetes on the development and progression of long-term complications of insulin-dependent diabetes mellitus. *N Engl J Med* 1993; 329: 977–86.

De Laet CEDH, Van Hout BA, Burger H, et al. Hip fracture prediction in elderly men and women: validation in the Rotterdam Study. *J Bone Miner Res* 1998; 13: 1587–93.

De Smet PAGM. Herbal remedies. *N Engl J Med* 2002; 347: 2046–56.

Diabetes Prevention Program Research Group. Reduction in the incidence of type 2 diabetes with lifestyle intervention or metformin. *N Engl J Med* 2002; 346: 393–403.

Diez Roux AV, Merkin SS, Arnett D, et al. Neighborhood of residence and incidence of coronary heart disease. *N Engl J Med* 2001; 345: 99–106.

Djulbegovic B, Lacevic M, Cantor A, et al. The uncertainty principle and industry-sponsored research. *Lancet* 2000; 356: 635–8.

Drazen JM. Inappropriate advertising of dietary supplements. *N Engl J Med* 2003; 348: 777–8.

Drazen JM, Curfman GD. Financial associations of authors. *N Engl J Med* 2002; 346: 1901–2.

Druss BG, Marcus SC, Olfson M, et al. Trends in care by nonphysician clinicians in the United States. *N Engl J Med* 2003; 348: 130–7.

Eastham JA, Riedel E, Scardino PT, et al. Variation of serum prostate-specific-antigen levels. *JAMA* 2003; 289: 2695–700.

Edmond SL, Felson DT. Prevalence of back symptoms in elders. *J Rheumatol* 2000; 27: 220–5.

Edwards A, Unigwe S, Elwyn G, Hood K. Effects of communicating individual risks in screening programmes: Cochrane systematic review. *BMJ* 2003; 327: 703–9.

Elmore JG, Barton MB, Moceri VM, et al. Ten-year risk of false positive screening mammograms and clinical breast examinations. *N Engl J Med* 1998; 338: 1089–96.

Elmore JG, Wells C, Lee CH, et al. Variability in radiologists' interpretations of mammograms. *N Engl J Med* 1994; 331: 1493–9.

Engelhart MJ, Geerlings MI, Ruitenberg A, et al. Dietary intake of antioxidants and risk of Alzheimer disease. *JAMA* 2002; 287: 3223–9.

Ensrud KE, Duong T, Cauley JA, et al. Low fractional calcium absorption increases the risk for hip fracture in women with low calcium intake. *Ann Intern Med* 2000; 132: 345–53.

Erichsen JE. *Railway and Other Injuries of the Nervous System.* London: Walton and Maberly, 1866.

Ernst E. The risk-benefit profile of commonly used herbal therapies: ginkgo, St John's wort, ginseng, echinacea, saw palmetto, and kava. *Ann Intern Med* 2002; 136: 42–53.

Ernst E. Herbal medicines put into context. *BMJ* 2003; 327: 881–2.

Ettinger B, Black DM, Mitlak BH, et al. Reduction of vertebral fracture risk in postmenopausal women with osteoporosis treated with raloxifene. *JAMA* 1999; 282: 637–45.

Fairfield KM, Fletcher RH. Vitamins for chronic disease prevention in adults. *JAMA* 2002; 287: 3116–26.

Farmer JA. Learning from the cerivastatin experience. *Lancet* 2001; 358: 1383–5.

Fawzi W, Stampfer MJ. A role for multivitamins in infection? *Ann Intern Med* 2003; 138: 430–1.

Felson DT, McAlindon TE. Glucosamine and chondroitin for osteoarthritis: to recommend or not to recommend? *Arthritis Care Res* 2000; 13: 179–82.

Ferrie JE, Shipley MJ, Marmot MG, Stansfeld SA, Davey Smith G. An uncertain future: the health effects of threats to employment security in white-collar men and women. *Am J Public Health* 1998; 88: 1030–6.

Feskanich D, Willett W, Colditz G. Walking and leisure-time activity and risk of hip fracture in postmenopausal women. *JAMA* 2002; 288: 2300–6.

Finkler K. *Experiencing the New Genetics.* Philadelphia: University of Pennsylvania Press, 2000.

Fischoff B, Wesseley S. Managing patients with inexplicable health problems. *BMJ* 2003; 326: 595–7.

Fisher B, Anderson S, Bryant J, et al. Twenty-year follow-up of a randomized trial comparing total mastectomy, lumpectomy, and lumpectomy plus irradiation for the treatment of invasive breast cancer. *N Engl J Med* 2002; 347: 1233–41.

Fisher B, Jeong J-H, Anderson S, et al. Twenty-five-year follow-up of a randomized trial comparing radical mastectomy, total mastectomy, and total mastectomy followed by irradiation. *N Engl J Med* 2002; 347: 567–75.

Fisher B, Redmond C, Fisher ER, et al. Ten-year results of a randomized clinical trial comparing radical mastectomy and total mastectomy with or without radiation. *N Engl J Med* 1985; 312: 674–81.

Fisher ES, Wennberg DE, Stukel TA, et al. The implications of regional variations in Medicare spending. Part 1: The content, quality, and accessibility of care. *Ann Intern Med* 2003; 138: 273–87.

Fisher ES, Wennberg DE, Stukel TA, et al. The implications of regional variations in Medicare spending. Part 2: Health outcomes and satisfaction with care. *Ann Intern Med* 2003; 138: 288–98.

Fitzpatrick R. Social status and mortality. *Ann Intern Med* 2001; 134: 1001–3.

Fletcher RH. Screening sigmoidoscopy – how often and how good? *JAMA* 2003; 290: 106–8.

Fletcher S, Colditz G. Failure of estrogen plus progestin therapy for prevention. *JAMA* 2002; 288: 366–8.

Fletcher S, Elmore JG. Mammographic screening for breast cancer. *N Engl J Med* 2003; 348: 1672–80.

Foley DJ, White LR. Dietary intake of antioxidants and risk of Alzheimer disease. *JAMA* 2002; 287: 3261–3.

Fonseca R, Hartmann LC, Petersen IV, et al. Ductal carcinoma in situ of the breast. *Ann Intern Med* 1997; 127: 1013–22.

Fontanarosa PB, Rennie D, DeAngelis CD. The need for regulation of dietary supplements – lessons from ephedra. *JAMA* 2003; 289: 1568–70.

Ford ES, Giles WH, Dietz WH. Prevalence of the metabolic syndrome among US adults. *JAMA* 2002; 287: 356–9.

Forseth KØ, Husby G, Gran JT, Førre Ø. Prognostic factors for the development of fibromyalgia in women with self-reported musculoskeletal pain: a prospective study. *J Rheumatol* 1999; 26: 2458–67.

Foucault M. *The Birth of the Clinic: An Archaeology of Medical Perception.* Trans. A Sheridan. London: Tavistock, 1973.

Fransen M, McConnell S, Bell M. Therapeutic exercise for people with osteoarthritis of the hip or knee: a systematic review. *J Rheumatol* 2002; 29: 1737–45.

Frazier AL, Colditz GA, Fuchs CS, Kuntz KM. Cost-effectiveness of screening for colorectal cancer in the general population. *JAMA* 2000; 284: 1954–61.

Freemantle N, Calvert M, Woods J, Eastaugh J, Griffin C. Composite outcomes in randomized trials. *JAMA* 2003; 289: 2554–9.

Freidson E. *Medical Work in America.* New Haven: Yale University Press, 1989.

Friedman HS. Coronary bypass graft surgery: reexamining the assumptions. *J Gen Intern Med* 1990; 5: 80–3.

Furlan AD, Brosseau L, Imamura M, Irvin E. Massage for low-back pain: a systematic review within the framework of the Cochrane Collaboration Back Review Group. *Spine* 2002; 27: 1896–1910.

Gadamer H-G. *The Enigma of Health: The Art of Healing in a Scientific Age.* Trans. J Gaiger, N Walker. Stanford: Stanford University Press, 1996.

Gann PH, Morrow M. Combined hormone therapy and breast cancer. *JAMA* 2003; 290: 3304–6.

Garro LC. Chronic illness and the construction of narratives. In: Good M-J D, Brodwin PE, Good BJ, Kleinman A, eds. *Pain as Human Experience.* Berkeley: University of California Press, 1992: 100–37.

Gevitz N. Sectarian medicine. *JAMA* 1987; 257: 1636–40.

Gibson JNA, Grant IC, Waddell G. The Cochrane Review of surgery for lumbar disc prolapse and degenerative lumbar spondylosis. *Spine* 1999; 24: 1820–32.

Gillespie LD, Gillespie WJ, Cumming R, et al. Review: multiple risk factor modification reduces falls in elderly persons. In: *The Cochrane Database of Systematic Reviews.* The Cochrane Library. Oxford: Update Software; 1998, Issue 1.

Gøtzsche PC, Olsen O. Is screening for breast cancer with mammography justifiable? *Lancet* 2000; 355: 129–34.

Goldacre MJ, Roberts SE, Yeates D. Mortality after admission to hospital with fractured neck of femur: database study. *BMJ* 2002; 325: 868–9.

Goldberg RJ, Gore JM, Alpert JS, Dalen JE. Recent changes in attack and survival rates of acute myocardial infarction (1975–1981). *JAMA* 1986; 255: 2774–9.

Gomez-Marin O, Folsom AR, Kottke TE, et al. Improvement in the long-term survival among patients hospitalized with acute myocardial infarction, 1970–1980. *N Engl J Med* 1987; 21: 1354–9.

Goodman SN. The mammography dilemma: a crisis for evidence-based medicine? *Ann Intern Med* 2002; 137: 363–5.

Graat JM, Schouten EG, Kok FJ. Effect of daily vitamin E and multivitamin-mineral supplementation on acute respiratory tract infections in elderly persons. *JAMA* 2002; 288: 715–21.

Greenhalgh S. *Under the Medical Gaze: Facts and Fictions of Chronic Pain.* Berkeley: University of California Press, 2001.

Greenspan SL, Emkey RD, Bone HG, et al. Significant differential effects of alendronate, estrogen, or combination therapy on the rate of bone loss after discontinuation of treatment of postmenopausal osteoporosis. *Ann Intern Med* 2002; 137: 875–83.

Greenspan SL, Myers ER, Maitland LA, et al. Fall severity and bone mineral density as risk factors for hip fracture in ambulatory elderly. *JAMA* 1994; 271: 128–33.

Gregg EW, Cauley JA, Stone K, et al. Relationship of changes in physical acitivity and mortality among older women. *JAMA* 2003; 289: 2379–86.

Gregg EW, Gerzoff RB, Thompson TJ, Williamson DF. Intentional weight loss and death in overweight and obese US adults 35 years of age and older. *Ann Intern Med* 2003; 138: 383–9.

Grodstein F, Clarkson TB, Manson JE. Understanding the divergent data on postmenopausal hormone therapy. *N Engl J Med* 2003; 348: 645–50.

Guastello SJ, Johnson EA, Rieke ML. Nonlinear dynamics of motivational flow. *Nonlinear Dynamics, Psychology, and Life Sciences* 1999; 3: 259–73.

Gureje O, von Korff M, Simon GE, Gater R. Persistent pain and well-being: a World Health Organization study in primary care. *JAMA* 1998; 280: 147–51.

Gurwitz JH, Field TS, Harrold LR, et al. Incidence and preventability of adverse drug events among older persons in the ambulatory setting. *JAMA* 2003; 289: 1107–16.

Hacohen M. *Karl Popper: The Formative Years 1902–1945*. Cambridge: Cambridge University Press, 2000.

Hacking I. *The Social Construction of What?* Cambridge: Harvard University Press, 2000.

Hadler NM. There's the forest: the object lesson of NSAID gastropathy. *J Rheumatol* 1990; 17: 280–2.

Hadler NM. Knee pain is the malady – not osteoarthritis. *Ann Intern Med* 1992; 116: 598–9.

Hadler NM. The injured worker and the internist. *Ann Intern Med* 1994; 120: 163–4.

Hadler NM. If you have to prove you are ill, you can't get well: the object lesson of fibromyalgia. *Spine* 1996; 21: 2397–400.

Hadler NM. Workers' compensation and chronic regional musculoskeletal pain. *Brit J Rheumatol* 1998; 37: 815–8.

Hadler NM. Laboring for longevity. *J Occup Environ Med* 1999; 41: 617–21.

Hadler NM. Back pain. Chapter 13.2. In: Evans JG, Williams TF, Beattie BL, Michel J-P, Wilcock GK, eds. *Oxford Textbook of Geriatric Medicine*. 2nd ed. Oxford: Oxford University Press, 2000: 559–65.

Hadler NM. Chiropractic. *Rheum Dis Clin of North Am* 2000; 26: 97–102.

Hadler NM. The "ergonomics injury" as a social construction. *Workers' Compensation Policy Review* 2001; 1: 20–5.

Hadler NM. Rheumatology and the health of the workforce. *Arthritis Rheum* 2001; 44: 1971–4.

Hadler NM. Options in disability determination: lessons that pertain to the regional musculoskeletal disorders. *J Rheumatol* 2002; 29: 407–10.

Hadler NM. Point of view on the paper by Coulter et al. *Spine* 2002; 27: 297–8.

Hadler NM. A ripe old age. *Arch Intern Med* 2003; 163: 1261–2.

Hadler NM. "Fibromyalgia" and the medicalization of misery. *J Rheumatol* 2003; 30: 1668–70.

Hadler NM. MRI for regional back pain: need for less imaging, better understanding. *JAMA* 2003; 289: 2863–5.

Hadler NM. The semiotics of "upper limb musculoskeletal disorders in workers." *J Clin Epidemiol* 2003; 56: 937–9.

Hadler NM. *Occupational Musculoskeletal Disorders.* 3rd ed. Philadelphia: Lippincott Williams & Wilkins, 2004.

Hadler NM, Curtis P, Gillings DB, Stinnett S. A benefit of spinal manipulation as adjunctive therapy for acute low back pain: a stratified controlled trial. *Spine* 1987; 12: 703–6.

Hadler NM, Evans JP. Commentary on "The Kin in the Gene." *Current Anthropology* 2001; 42: 252–3.

Hadler NM, Gillings DB. On the design of the phase III drug trial. *Arthritis Rheum* 1983; 26: 1354–61.

Hagen KB, Hilde G, Jamtvedt G, Winnem MF. The Cochrane Review of advice to stay active as a single treatment for low back pain and sciatica. *Spine* 2002: 27: 1736–41.

Hajjar I, Kotchen TA. Trends in prevalence, awareness, treatment and control of hypertension in the United States, 1988–2000. *JAMA* 2003; 290: 199–206.

Haller CA, Benowitz NL. Adverse cardiovascular and central nervous system events associated with dietary supplements containing ephedra alkaloids. *N Engl J Med* 2000; 343: 1833–8.

Hanger HC, Smart EJ, Marrilees MJ, Frampton CM. The prevalence of malnutrition in elderly hip fracture patients. *NZ Med J* 1999; 112: 88–90.

Hannan EL, Magaziner J, Wang JJ, et al. Mortality and locomotion 6 months after hospitalization for hip fracture. *JAMA* 2001; 285: 2736–42.

Hannan EL, Racz MJ, Walford G, et al. Predictors of readmission for complications of coronary artery bypass graft surgery. *JAMA* 2003; 290: 773–80.

Harris R, Lohr KN. Screening for prostate cancer: an update of the evidence for the us Preventive Services Task Force. *Ann Intern Med* 2002; 137: 917–29.

Harris ST, Watts NB, Genant HK, et al. Effects of risedronate treatment on vertebral and nonvertebral fractures in women with postmenopausal osteoporosis. *JAMA* 1999; 282: 1344–52.

Hassett AL, Cone JD, Patella SJ, Sigal LH. The role of catastrophizing in the pain and depression of women with fibromyalgia syndrome. *Arthritis Rheum* 2000; 43: 2493–500.

Hays J, Ockene JK, Brunner RL, et al. Effects of estrogen plus progestin on health-related quality of life. *N Engl J Med* 2003; 348: 1839–54.

He K, Merchant A, Rimm EB, et al. Dietary fat intake and risk of stroke in male US healthcare professionals: 14 year prospective cohort study. *BMJ* 2003; 327: 777–81.

Heart Outcomes Prevention Evaluation Study Investigators. Vitamin E supplementation and cardiovascular events in high-risk patients. *N Engl J Med* 2000; 342: 154–60.

Hemingway H, Crook AM, Feder G, et al. Underuse of coronary revascularization procedures in patients considered appropriate candidates for revascularization. *N Engl J Med* 2001; 344: 645–54.

Hemingway H, Shipley M, Britton A, Page M, Macfarlane P, Marmot M. Prognosis of angina with and without a diagnosis: 11 year follow up in the Whitehall II prospective cohort study. *BMJ* 2003; 327: 895–99.

Hemingway H, Shipley MJ, Stansfeld S, Marmot M. Sickness absence from back pain, psychosocial work characteristics and employment grade among office workers. *Scand J Work Environ Health* 1997; 23: 121–9.

Herman J. Reflections on playing God engendered by a chat with L. *Perspectives Biol Med* 1993; 36: 592–5.

Hertzman C. Health and human society. *American Scientist* 2001; 89: 538–45.

Hertzman-Miller RR, Morgenstern H, Hurwitz EL, et al. Comparing the satisfaction of low back pain patients randomized to receive medical or chiropractic care: results from the UCLA low-back pain study. *Am J Public Health* 2002; 92: 1628–33.

Hlatky M. Patient preferences and clinical guidelines. *JAMA* 1995; 273: 1219–20.

Hlatky MA, Boothroyd D, Vittinghoff E, et al. Quality-of-life and depressive symptoms in postmenopausal women after receiving hormone therapy. *JAMA* 2002; 287: 591–7.

Hoes AW, Grobbee DE, Lubsen J, et al. Diuretics, ß-blockers, and the risk for sudden cardiac death in hypertensive patients. *Ann Intern Med* 1995; 123: 481–7.

Holmberg L, Bill-Axelson A, Helgesen F, et al. A randomized trial comparing radical prostatectomy with watchful waiting in early prostate cancer. *N Engl J Med* 2002; 347: 781–9.

Holmes OW. *Medical Essays: 1842–1882*. Boston: Houghton Mifflin, 1899.

Hoogendoorn WE, van Poppel MNM, Bongers PM, et al. Systematic review of psychosocial factors at work and private life as risk factors for back pain. *Spine* 2000; 25: 2114–25.

Hoving JL, Gross AR, Gasner D, et al. A critical appraisal of review articles on the effectiveness of conservative treatment for neck pain. *Spine* 2001; 26: 196–205.

Hu FB, Bronner L, Willett WC, et al. Fish and omega-3 fatty acid intake and risk of coronary heart disease in women. *JAMA* 2002; 287: 1815–21.

Hu FB, Stampfer MJ, Rimm EB, et al. A prospective study of egg consumption and risk of cardiovascular disease in men and women. *JAMA* 1999; 281: 1387–94.

Humphrey LL, Chan GKS, Sox HC. Postmenopausal hormone replacement therapy and the primary prevention of cardiovascular disease. *Ann Intern Med* 2002; 137: 273–84.

Humphrey LL, Helfand M, Chan BKS, Woolf SH. Breast cancer screening: a summary of the evidence for the US Preventive Services Task Force. *Ann Intern Med* 2002; 137: 347–60.

Hunt, IM, Silman, AJ, Benjamin, S, et al. The prevalence and associated features of chronic widespread pain in the community using the "Manchester" definition of chronic widespread pain. *Rheumatology* 1999; 38: 275–9.

Imperiale TF. Aspirin and the prevention of colorectal cancer. *N Engl J Med* 2003; 348: 879–80.

Imperiale TF, Wagner DR, Lin CY, et al. Results of screening colonoscopy among persons 40 to 49 years of age. *N Engl J Med* 2002; 346: 1781–5.

Irnich D, Beharens N, Molzen H, et al. Randomised trial of acupuncture compared with conventional massage and "sham" laser acupuncture for treatment of chronic neck pain. *BMJ* 2001; 322: 1574–8.

Jackson SA, Tenenhouse A, Robertson L, et al. Vertebral fracture definition from population-based data: preliminary results from the Canadian Multicentre Osteoporosis Study (CaMos). *Osteoporos Int* 2000; 11: 680–7.

Jacobs AK. Primary angioplasty for acute myocardial infarction – is it worth the wait? *N Engl J Med* 2003; 349: 798–800.

Jha P, Flather M, Lonn E, et al. The antioxidant vitamins and cardio-vascular disease: a critical review of epidemiologic and clinical trial data. *Ann Intern Med* 1995; 123: 860–72.

Johnston JM, Landsittel DP, Nelson NA, et al. Stressful psychosocial work environment increases risk for back pain among retail material handlers. *Am J Ind Med* 2003; 43: 179–87.

Johnstone RT. *Occupational Diseases: Diagnosis, Medicolegal Aspects and Treatment.* Philadelphia: Saunders, 1941.

Joines JD, Hadler NM. Back pain. Chapter 100. In: Wachter RM, Goldman L, Hollander H, eds. *Hospital Medicine.* Philadelphia: Lippincott Williams & Wilkins, 2000: 961–8.

Jonas WB, Kaptchuk TJ, Linde K. A critical overview of homeopathy. *Ann Intern Med* 2003; 138: 393–9.

Jüni P, Rutjes AWS, Dieppe PA. Are selective COX 2 inhibitors superior to traditional non-steroidal anti-inflammatory durgs? *BMJ* 2002; 324: 1287–8.

Kalb PE, Koehler KG. Legal issues in scientific research. *JAMA* 2002; 287: 85–91.

Kannus P, Parkkari J, Koskinen S, et al. Fall-induced injuries and deaths among older adults. *JAMA* 1999; 281: 1895–9.

Kannus P, Parkkari J, Niemi S, et al. Prevention of hip fracture in elderly people with use of a hip protector. *N Engl J Med* 2000; 343: 1506–13.

Kaplan JB, Bennett T. Use of race and ethnicity in biomedical publication. *JAMA* 2003; 289: 2709–16.

Kaptchuk TJ. The placebo effect in alternative medicine: can the performance of a healing ritual have clinical significance? *Ann Intern Med* 2002; 136: 817–25.

Kaptchuk TJ. Effect of interpretive bias on research evidence. *BMJ* 2003; 326: 1453–5.

Kaptchuk TJ, Eisenberg DM. The persuasive appeal of alternative medicine. *Ann Intern Med* 1998; 129: 1061–5.

Karasek RA, Theorell T. *Healthy Work.* New York: Basic Books, 1990.

Katz JN. Patient preferences and health disparities. *JAMA* 2001; 286: 1506–8.

Kaufman M. Homeopathy in America: the rise and fall and persistence of a medical heresy. In: Gevitz N, ed. *Other Healers: Unorthodox Medicine in America*. Baltimore: Johns Hopkins University Press, 1988: 99–123.

Kawachi I, Berkman LF, eds. *Neighborhoods and Health*. New York: Oxford University Press, 2003.

Kawachi I, Kennedy BP, Wilkinson RG, eds. *The Society and Population Health Reader.* Vol. 1: *Income Inequality and Health*. New York: The New Press, 1999.

Kelch RP. Maintaining the public trust in clinical research. *N Engl J Med* 2002; 346: 285–7.

Keller T, Chappell T. The rise and fall of Erichsen's disease (railway spine). *Spine* 1996; 21: 1597–601.

Kersh BC, Bradley LA, Alarcón GS, et al. Psychosocial and health status variables independently predict health care seeking in fibromyalgia. *Arthritis Care Res* 2001; 45: 362–71.

King SB. Why have stents replaced balloons? underwhelming evidence. *Ann Intern Med* 2003; 138: 842–3.

Kjaergard LL, Als-Nielsen B. Associations between competing interests and authors' conclusions: epidemiological study of randomized clinical trials published in the *BMJ*. *BMJ* 2002; 325: 249–52.

Klauokalani D, Sherman KJ, Cherkin DC. Acupuncture for chronic low back pain: diagnosis and treatment patterns among acupuncturists evaluating the same patient. *South Med J* 2001; 94: 486–92.

Koes BW, Assendelft WJ, van der Heijden GJ, Bouter LM. Spinal manipulation for low back pain: an updated systematic review of randomized clinical trials. *Spine* 1996; 21: 2860–71.

Korn D. Conflicts of interest in biomedical research. *JAMA* 2000; 284: 2234–7.

Krzyzanowska MK, Pintilie M, Tannock IF. Factors associated with failure to publish large randomized trials presented at an oncology meeting. *JAMA* 2003; 290: 495–501.

Kubzansky LD, Kawachi I, Sparrow D. Socioeconomic status, hostility, and risk factor clustering in the normative aging study: any help from the concept of allostatic load? *Ann Behav Med* 1999; 21: 330–8.

Kuhn T. *The Structure of Scientific Revolutions*. 2nd ed. Chicago: University of Chicago Press, 1970.

Kumana CR, Cheung BMY, Lauder IJ. Gauging the impact of statins using number needed to treat. *JAMA* 1999; 282: 1899–901.

Laine L, Wogen J, Yu H. Gastrointestinal health care resource utilization with chronic use of COX-2-specific inhibitors versus traditional NSAIDS. *Gastroenterology* 2003; 125: 389–95.

Lakka H-M, Laaksonen DE, Lakka TA, et al. The metabolic syndrome and total and cardiovascular disease mortality in middle-aged men. *JAMA* 2002; 288: 2709–16.

Lakka TA, Venäläinen JM, Rauramaa R, et al. Relation of leisure-time physical activity and cardiorespiratory fitness to the risk of acute myocardial infarction in men. *N Engl J Med* 1994; 330: 1549–54.

Lantz PM, House JS, Lepkowski JM, et al. Socioeconomic factors, health behaviors, and mortality. *JAMA* 1998; 279: 1703–8.

Lasser KE, Allen PD, Woolhandler SJ, et al. Timing of new black box warnings and withdrawals for prescription medications. *JAMA* 2002; 287: 2215–20.

Lauer MS, Topol EJ. Clinical trials – multiple treatments, multiple end points, and multiple lessons. *JAMA* 2003; 289: 2575–7.

Lavizzo-Mourey R, Knickman JR. Racial disparities – the need for research and action. *N Engl J Med* 2003; 349: 1379–80.

Law MR, Wald NJ, Morris JK, Jordan RE. Value of low dose combination treatment with blood pressure lowering drugs: analysis of 354 randomised trials. *BMJ* 2003; 326: 1427–35.

LeBoff MS, Kohlmeier L, Hurwitz S, Franklin J, Wright J, Glowacki J. Occult vitamin D deficiency in postmenopausal women with acute hip fracture. *JAMA* 1999; 281: 1505–11.

Leeb BF, Schweitzer H, Montag K, Smolen JS. A meta-analysis of chondroitin sulfate in the treatment of osteoarthritis. *J Rheumatol* 2000; 27: 205–11.

Leipzig RM, Cumming RG, Tinetti ME. Drugs and falls in older people: a systematic review and meta-analysis: II. Cardiac and analgesic drugs. *J Am Geriatr Soc* 1999; 47: 40–50.

Lerman C, Trock B, Rimer BK, et al. Psychological and behavioral implications of abnormal mammograms. *Ann Intern Med* 1991; 114: 657–61.

Lerner BH. Fighting the war on breast cancer: debates over early detection, 1945 to the present. *Ann Intern Med* 1998; 129: 74–8.

Levy D, Thom TJ. Death rates from coronary disease – progress and a puzzling paradox. *N Engl J Med* 1998; 339: 915–7.

Lexchin J, Bero LA, Djulbegovic B, Clark O. Pharmaceutical industry sponsorship and research outcome and quality: systematic review. *BMJ* 2003; 326: 1167–77.

Lieberman DA, Weiss DG, for the Veterans Affairs Cooperative Study Group. One-time screening for colorectal cancer with combined fecal occult-blood testing and examination of the distal colon. *N Engl J Med* 2001; 345: 555–60.

Lieberman DA, Weiss DG, Bond JH, et al. Use of colonoscopy to screen asymptomatic adults for colorectal cancer. *N Engl J Med* 2000; 343: 162–8.

Linde K, Mulrow CD. St. John's wort for depression. *Cochrane Review,* Cochrane Library, Oxford: Update Software, 1998.

Lindsay R, Silverman SL, Cooper C, et al. Risk of new vertebral fracture in the year following a fracture. *JAMA* 2001; 285: 320–3.

Linton SJ. A review of psychological risk factors in back and neck pain. *Spine* 2000; 25: 1148–56.

Linton SJ, Van Tulder MW. Preventive interventions for back and neck pain problems: what is the evidence? *Spine* 2001; 26: 778–87.

Lips P. Hypervitaminosis A and fractures. *N Engl J Med* 2003; 348: 347–9.

Lipsky PE, Abramson SB, Breedveld FC, et al. Analysis of the effect of cox-2 specific inhibitors and recommendations for their use in clinical practice. *J Rheumatol* 2000; 27: 1338–40.

Lucire Y. *Constructing RSI: Belief and Desire.* Sydney: University of New South Wales Press, 2003.

Lu-Yao G, Albertsen PC, Stanford JL, et al. Natural experiment examining impact of aggressive screening and treatment on prostate cancer mortality in two fixed cohorts from Seattle area and Connecticut. *BMJ* 2002; 325: 740–3.

Lynch HT, de la Chapelle A. Hereditary colorectal cancer. *N Engl J Med* 2003; 348: 919–32.

Macfarlane GJ, Morris S, Hunt IM, et al. Chronic widespread pain in the community: the influence of psychological symptoms and mental disorder on healthcare seeking behavior. *J Rheumatol* 1999; 26: 413–9.

Macfarlane GJ, Thomas E, Papageorgiou AC, et al. The natural history of chronic pain in the community: a better prognosis than in the clinic? *J Rheumatol* 1996; 23: 1617–20.

Mahoney EM, Jurkovitz CT, Chu H, et al. Cost and cost-effectiveness of an early invasive vs conservative strategy for the treatment of unstable angina and non-ST-segment elevation myocardial infarction. *JAMA* 2002; 288: 1851–8.

Main CJ, Williams AC. Musculoskeletal pain. *BMJ* 2002; 325: 534–7.

Mandel JS, Bond JH, Church TR, et al. Reducing mortality from colorectal cancer by screening for fecal occult blood. *N Engl J Med* 1993; 328: 1365–71.

Mandel JS, Church TR, Bond JH, et al. The effect of fecal occult-blood screening on the incidence of colorectal cancer. *N Engl J Med* 2000; 343: 1603–7.

Mann CC, Plummer ML. *The Aspirin Wars.* New York: Knopf, 1991.

Manson JE, Hsia J, Johnson KC, et al. Estrogen plus progestin and the risk of coronary heart disease. *N Engl J Med* 2003; 349: 523–34.

March LM, Cameron ID, Cumming RG, et al. Mortality and morbidity after hip fracture: can evidence based clinical pathways make a difference? *J Rheumatol* 2000; 27: 2227–31.

Marcus AJ, Broekman MJ, Pinsky DJ. cox inhibitors and thrombophilia. *N Engl J Med* 2002; 347: 1025–6.

Marcus DM, Grollman AP. Botanical medicines – the need for new regulations. *N Engl J Med* 2002; 347: 2073–6.

Mark DB, Newman MF. Protecting the brain in coronary artery bypass graft surgery. *JAMA* 2002; 287: 1448–50.

Marmot M, Wilkinson RH, eds. *Social Determinants of Health.* Oxford: Oxford University Press, 1999.

Marra CA, Esdaile JM, Sun H, Anis AH. The cost of cox inhibitors: how selective should we be? *J Rheumatol* 2000; 27: 2731–3.

Masud T, Francis RM. The increasing use of peripheral bone densitometry. *BMJ* 2000; 321: 306–8.

McAlindon TE, LaValley MP, Gulin JP, Felson DT. Glucosamine and chondroitin for treatment of osteoarthritis: a systematic quality assessment and meta-analysis. *JAMA* 2000; 283: 1469–75.

McCally M, Haines A, Fein O, et al. Poverty and ill health: physicians can, and should, make a difference. *Ann Intern Med* 1998; 129: 726–33.

McClung MR, Geusens P, Miller PD, et al. Effect of risedronate on the risk of hip fracture in elderly women. *N Engl J Med* 2001; 344: 333–40.

McDonald CJ. Medical heuristics: the silent adjudicators of clinical practice. *Ann Intern Med* 1996; 124: 56–62.

McGovern PG, Pankow JS, Shahar E, et al. Recent trends in acute coronary heart disease. *N Engl J Med* 1996; 334: 884–90.

McLeod RS and members of the Canadian Task Force on Preventive Health Care. Screening strategies for colorectal cancer: a systematic review of the evidence. *Can J Gastroenterol* 2001; 15:647–60.

McTigue KM, Garrett JM, Popkin BM. The natural history of the development of diabetes in a cohort of young US adults between 1981 and 1998. *Ann Intern Med* 2002; 136: 857–64.

McWhinney IR, Epstein RM, Freeman TR. Rethinking somatization. *Ann Intern Med* 1997; 126: 747–50.

Meeker WC, Haldeman S. Chiropractic: a profession at the crossroads of mainstream and alternative medicine. *Ann Intern Med* 2002; 136: 216–27.

Meigs JB. The metabolic syndrome. *BMJ* 2003; 327: 61–2.

Melander H, Ahlqvist-Rastad J, Meijer G, Beermann B. Evidence b(i)ased medicine – selective reporting from studies sponsored by pharmaceutical industry: review of studies in new drug applications. *BMJ* 2003; 326: 1171–6.

Michaëlsson K, Lithell H, Vessby B, Melhus H. Serum retinol levels and the risk of fracture. *N Engl J Med* 2003; 348: 287–94.

Miettinen OS, Henschke CI, Pasmantier MW, et al. Does mammography save lives? *Can Med Assoc J* 2002; 166: 1187–8.

Miettinen OS, Henschke CI, Pasmantier MW, et al. Mammographic screening: no reliable supporting evidence? *Lancet* 2002; 359: 404–6; *http://image.theLancet.com/extras/1093web.pdf*

Mikkelsson, M, Kaprio, J, Salminen, JJ, et al. Widespread pain among 11-year-old Finnish twin pairs. *Arthritis Rheum* 2001; 44: 481–5.

Miller AB, Baines CJ, To T, Wall C. Canadian National Breast Screening Study: 1. Breast cancer detection and death rates among women aged 40 to 49 years. *Can Med Assoc J* 1992; 147: 1459–76.

Miller AB, Baines CJ, To T, Wall C. Canadian National Breast Screening Study: 2. Breast cancer detection and death rates among women aged 50 to 59 years. *Can Med Assoc J* 1992; 147: 1477–88.

Miller AB, To T, Baines CJ, Wall C. Canadian National Breast Screening Study – 2: 13-year results of a randomized trial in women aged 50–59 years. *J Natl Cancer Inst* 2000; 92: 1490–9.

Miller AB, To T, Baines CJ, Wall C. The Canadian National Breast Screening Study – 1: Breast cancer mortality after 11 to 16 years of follow-up. *Ann Intern Med* 2002; 137: 305–12.

Miller D. *Popper Selections.* Princeton: Princeton University Press, 1985.

Miller FG, Rosenstein DL, DeRenzo EG. Professional integrity in clinical research. *JAMA* 1998; 280: 1449–54.

Mills JL. Data torturing. *N Engl J Med* 1993; 329: 1196–9.

Mixter WJ, Barr JS. Rupture of the intervertebral disc with involvement of the spinal canal. *N Engl J Med* 1934; 211: 210–5.

Mohren DCL, Swaen GMH, van Amelsvoort LGPM, et al. Job insecurity as a risk factor for common infections and health complaints. *J Occup Environ Med* 2003; 45: 123–9.

Morin K, Rakatansky H, Riddick FA, et al. Managing conflicts of interest in the conduct of clinical trials. *JAMA* 2002; 287: 78–84.

Morris CD, Carson S. Routine vitamin supplementation to prevent cardiovascular disease: a summary of the evidence for the us Preventive Services Task Force. *Ann Intern Med* 2003; 139: 56–70.

Morris MC, Evans DA, Bienias JL, et al. Dietary intake of antioxidant nutrients and the risk of incident Alzheimer disease in a biracial community study. *JAMA* 2002; 287: 3230–7.

Morrow M, Schnitt SJ. Treatment selection in ductal carcinoma in situ. *JAMA* 2000; 283: 453–5.

Mortality Morbidity Weekly Report (CDC) 1994; 43: 586.

Moseley JB, O'Malley K, Petersen NJ, et al. A controlled trial of arthroscopic surgery for osteoarthritis of the knee. *N Engl J Med* 2002; 347: 81–8.

Moses H, Braunwald E, Martin JB, Their SO. Collaborating with industry – choices for the academic medical center. *N Engl J Med* 2002; 347: 1371–5.

Mukherjee D, Nissen SE, Topol EJ. Risk of cardiovascular events associated with selective cox-2 inhibitors. *JAMA* 2001; 286: 954–9.

Multiple Risk Factor Intervention Trial Research Group. Multiple Risk Factor Intervention Trial: risk factor changes and mortality. *JAMA* 1982; 248: 182–7.

Musgrave DS, Vogt MT, Nevitt MC, Cauley JA. Back problems among postmenopausal women taking estrogen replacement therapy. *Spine* 2001; 26: 1606–12.

Narayan KMV, Boyle JP, Thompson TJ, Sorensen SW, Williamson DF. Lifetime risk for diabetes mellitus in the United States. *JAMA* 2003; 290: 1884–90.

National Cholesterol Education Program (NCEP). Executive summary of the third report on detection, evaluation and treatment of high blood cholesterol in adults. *JAMA* 2001; 285: 2486–97.

National Institutes of Health. Osteoporosis prevention, diagnosis and therapy. *NIH Consensus Statement* 2000; 17: 1–45.

National Institutes of Health. *Third Report of the National Cholesterol Education Program Expert Panel on Detection, Evaluation, and Treatment of High Blood Cholesterol in Adults (Adult Treatment Panel III).* Bethesda, MD: National Institutes of Health, 2001. NIH Publication 01–3670.

National Institutes of Health Consensus Development Panel on Osteoporosis Prevention, Diagnosis and Therapy. Osteoporosis prevention, diagnosis and therapy. *JAMA* 2001; 285: 785–95.

National Task Force on the Prevention and Treatment of Obesity. Weight cycling. *JAMA* 1994; 272: 1196–202.

Natvig B, Bruusgaard D, Eriksen W. Localized low back pain and low back pain as part of widespread musculoskeletal pain: two different disorders? a cross-sectional population study. *J Rehabil Med* 2001; 33: 21–5.

Neer RM, Arnaud CD, Zanchetta JR, et al. Effect of parathyroid hormone (1–34) on fractures and bone mineral density in postmenopausal women with osteoporosis. *N Engl J Med* 2001; 344: 1434–41.

Neerinckx J, van Houdenhove B, Lysens R, et al. Attributions in chronic fatigue syndrome and fibromyalgia syndrome in tertiary care. *J Rheumatol* 2000; 27: 1051–5.

Nelemans PJ, deBie RA, deVet HCW, Sturmans F. Injection therapy for subacute and chronic benign low back pain. *Spine* 2001; 26: 501–15.

Nelson HD, Helfand M, Woolf SH, Allan JD. Screening for postmenopausal osteoporosis: a review of the evidence for the US Preventive Services Task Force. *Ann Intern Med* 2002; 137: 529–41.

Nelson HD, Humphrey LL, Nygren P, et al. Postmenopausal hormone replacement therapy. *JAMA* 2002; 288: 872–81.

Nelson SP, Bärenholdt O, Diessel E, Armbrust S, Felsenberg D. Linearity and accuracy errors in bone densitometry. *Brit J Radiology* 1998; 71: 1062–8.

Nevitt MC, Ettinger B, Black DM, et al. The association of radiographically detected vertebral fractures with back pain and function: a prospective study. *Ann Intern Med* 1998; 128: 793–800.

Newman KS. *No Shame in My Game: The Working Poor in the Inner City.* New York: AA Knopf and The Russell Sage Foundation, 1999.

Newman MF, Kirchner JL, Phillips-Bute B, et al. Longitudinal assessment of neurocognitive function after coronary-artery bypass surgery. *N Engl J Med* 2001; 344: 395–402.

Nicassio PM, Weisman MH, Schuman C, Young CW. The role of generalized pain and pain behavior in tender point scores in fibromyalgia. *J Rheumatol* 2000; 27: 1056–62.

Nolan CM. Credibility, cookbook medicine, and common sense: guidelines and the College. *Ann Intern Med* 1994; 120: 966–7.

Nuovo J. Reporting number needed to treat and absolute risk reduction in randomized controlled trials. *JAMA* 2002; 287: 2813–4.

Olsen O, Gøtzsche PC. Cochrane review on screening for breast cancer with mammography. *Lancet* 2001; 358: 1340–2.

Orwoll E, Ettinger M, Weiss S, et al. Alendronate for the treatment of osteoporosis in men. *N Engl J Med* 2000; 343: 604–10.

Page DL, Jensen RA. Ductal carcinoma in situ of the breast. *JAMA* 1996; 275: 948–9.

Page DL, Simpson JF. Ductal carcinoma in situ – the focus for prevention, screening and breast conservation in breast cancer. *N Engl J Med* 1999; 340: 1499–500.

Pamuk E, Makuc D, Heck K, et al. *Socioeconomic Status and Health Chartbook: Health, United States, 1998.* Hyattsville, MD: National Center for Health Statistics, 1998.

Parker MJ, Gillespie LD, Gillespie WJ. Hip protectors for preventing hip fractures in the elderly. Cochrane Review, 1 May 1999. In: *The Cochrane Library.* Oxford: Update Software.

Passamani E, Davis KB, Gillespie MJ, Killip T, and the CASS Principal Investigators and Their Associates. A randomized trial of coronary artery bypass surgery: survival of patients with a low ejection fraction. *N Engl J Med* 1985; 312: 1665–71.

Pasternak RC. The ALLHAT lipid lowering trial – less is less. *JAMA* 2002; 288: 3042–4.

Payer L. *Medicine and Culture.* New York: Holt, 1988: 139–43.

Pell S, Fayerweather WE. Trends in the incidence of myocardial infarction and in associated mortality and morbidity in a large employed population 1957–1983. *N Engl J Med* 1985; 16: 1005–11.

Pendleton A, Arden N, Dougados M, et al. EULAR recommendations for the management of knee osteoarthritis: report of a task force of the Standing Committee for International Clinical Studies Including Therapeutic Trials (ESCISIT). *Ann Rheum Dis* 2000; 59: 936–44.

Perry HM, Davis BR, Price TR, et al. Effect of treating isolated systolic hypertension on the risk of developing various types and subtypes of stroke. *JAMA* 2000; 284: 465–71.

Pfisterer M, Buser P, Osswald S, et al. Outcome of elderly patients with chronic symptomatic coronary artery disease with an invasive vs optimized medical treatment strategy. *JAMA* 2003; 289: 1117–23.

Phillips K-A, Glendon G, Knight JA. Putting the risk of breast cancer in perspective. *N Engl J Med* 1999; 340: 141–4.

Phillips PS, Haas RH, Bannykh S, et al. Statin-associated myopathy with normal creatine kinase levels. *Ann Intern Med* 2002; 137: 581–5.

Pignone M, Phillips C, Mulrow C. Use of lipid lowering drugs for primary prevention of coronary heart disease: meta-analysis of randomized trials. *BMJ* 2000; 321: 983–6.

Pignone M, Saha S, Heorger T, Mandelblatt J. Cost-effectiveness analyses of colorectal cancer screening: a systematic review for the US Preventive Services Task Force. *Ann Intern Med* 2002; 137: 96–104.

Pincus T, Burton AK, Vogel S, Field AP. A systematic review of psychological factors as predictors of chronicity/disability in prospective cohorts of low back pain. *Spine* 2002; 27: E109–E120.

Podolsky DK. Going the distance – the case for true colorectal-cancer screening. *N Engl J Med* 2000; 343: 207–8.

Popper K. *Conjectures and Refutations.* London: Routledge, 2000.

Premier Collaborative Research Group. Effects of comprehensive lifestyle modification on blood pressure control. *JAMA* 2003; 289: 2083–93.

Price JR, Couper J. Cognitive behaviour therapy for adults with chronic fatigue syndrome. Cohcrane Review, 24 August 1998. In: *The Cochrane Library.* Oxford: Update software.

Psaty BM, Lumley T, Furberg CD, et al. Health outcomes associated with various antihypertensive therapies used as first-line agents. *JAMA* 2003; 289: 2534–44.

Psaty BM, Weiss NS, Furberg CD, et al. Surrogate end points, health outcomes, and the drug-approval process for the treatment of risk factors for cardiovascular disease. *JAMA* 1999; 282: 786–90.

Ransohoff DF, Collins MM, Fowler FJ. Why is prostate cancer screening so common when the evidence is so uncertain? a system without negative feedback. *Am J Med* 2002; 113: 663–7.

Ransohoff DF, Sandler RS. Screening for colorectal cancer. *N Engl J Med* 2002; 346: 40–4.

Rapp SR, Espeland MA, Shumaker SA, et al. Effect of estrogen plus progestin on global cognitive function in postmenopausal women. *JAMA* 2003; 289: 2663–72.

Ray WA, Stein CM, Daugherty JR, et al. cox-2 selective non-steroidal anti-inflammatory drugs and risk of serious coronary heart disease. *Lancet* 2002; 360: 1071–3.

Reaven GM. Importance of identifying the overweight patient who will benefit the most by losing weight. *Ann Intern Med* 2003; 138: 420–3.

Reid IR, Brown JP, Burckhardt P, et al. Intravenous zoledronic acid in postmenopausal women with low bone mineral density. *N Engl J Med* 2002: 346: 653–61.

Reissman DB, Orris P, Lacey R, Hartman DE. Downsizing, role demands, and job stress. *J Occup Environ Med* 1999; 41: 289–93.

Rekola KE, Levoska S, Takala J, Keinänen-Kiukaanniemi S. Patients with neck and shoulder complaints and multisite musculoskeletal symptoms – a prospective study. *J Rheumatol* 1997; 24: 2424–8.

Relman AS. Dealing with conflicts of interest. *N Engl J Med* 1984; 310: 1182–3.

Relman AS. New "information for authors" – and readers. *N Engl J Med* 1990; 323: 56.

Relman AS. Separating continuing medical education from pharmaceutical marketing. *JAMA* 2001; 285: 2009–12.

Relman AS. Financial associations of authors. *N Engl J Med* 2002; 347: 1043.

Relman AS. Defending professional independence. *JAMA* 2003; 289: 2418–20.

Rennie D, Luft HS. Pharmacoeconomic analyses. Making them transparent, making them credible. *JAMA* 2000; 283: 2158–60.

Rex DK, Cutler CS, Lemmel GT, et al. Colonoscopic miss rates of adenomas determined by back-to-back colonoscopies. *Gastroenterology* 1997: 112: 24–8.

Rey R. *The History of Pain.* Cambridge, MA: Harvard University Press, 1995.

Riggs BL, Hartmann LC. Selective estrogen-receptor modulators – mechanisms of action and application to clinical practice. *N Engl J Med* 2003; 348: 618–29.

Rimm EB, Ascherio A, Giovannucci E, et al. Vegetable, fruit and cereal fiber intake and risk of coronary heart disease among men. *JAMA* 1996; 275: 447–51.

RITA-2 trial participants. Coronary angioplasty versus medical therapy for angina: the second Randomised Intervention Treatment of Angina (RITA-2). *Lancet* 1997; 350: 461–8.

Roberts SE, Goldacre MJ. Time trends and demography of mortality after fractured neck of femur in an English population, 1968–98 database study. *BMJ* 2003; 327: 771–5.

Roos H, Laurén M, Adalberth T, et al. Knee osteoarthritis after meniscectomy. *Arthritis Rheum* 1998; 41: 687–93.

Rosa L, Rosa E, Sarner L, Barrett S. A close look at therapeutic touch. *JAMA* 1998; 279: 1005–10.

Rosamond WD, Chambless LE, Folsom AR, et al. Trends in the incidence of myocardial infarction and in mortality due to coronary heart disease, 1987–1994. *N Engl J Med* 1998; 339: 861–7.

Rosenthal MB, Berndt ER, Donohue JM, et al. Promotion of prescription drugs to consumers. *N Engl J Med* 2002; 346: 498–505.

Rothman K. *Causal Inference.* Cambridge: Epidemiology Resources, 1988.

Rubenstein LZ. Hip protectors – a breakthrough in fracture prevention. *N Engl J Med* 2000; 343: 1562–3.

Rubenstein LZ, Josephson KR, Trueblood PR, et al. Effects of a group exercise program on strength mobility and falls among fall-prone elderly men. *J Gerontol* 2000; 55A: M317–21.

Salkeld G, Cameron ID, Cumming RG, et al. Quality of life related to fear of falling and hip fracture in older women: a time trade off study. *BMJ* 2000; 320: 241–6.

Sandler RS, Halabi S, Baron JA, et al. A randomized trial of aspirin to prevent colorectal adenomas in patients with previous colorectal cancer. *N Engl J Med* 2003; 348: 883–90.

Satariano WA, Ragland DR. The effect of comorbidity on 3-year survival of women with primary breast cancer. *Ann Intern Med* 1994; 120: 104–10.

Scardino PT. The prevention of prostate cancer – the dilemma continues. *N Engl J Med* 2003; 349: 297–300.

Scarry E. *The Body in Pain*. New York: Oxford University Press, 1985.

Schnyder G, Roffi M, Flammer Y, Pin R, Hess OM. Effect of homocysteine-lowering therapy with folic acid, vitamin B_{12}, and vitamin B_6 on clinical outcome after percutaneous coronary intervention. *JAMA* 2002; 288: 973–9.

Schoen RE, Pinsky PF, Weissfeld JL, et al. Results of repeat sigmoidoscopy 3 years after a negative examination. *JAMA* 2003; 290: 41–8.

Schoenbaum SC. Toward fewer procedures and better outcomes. *JAMA* 1993; 269: 794–6.

Scholten RJ, Devillé WL, Opstelten W, et al. The accuracy of physical diagnostic tests for assessing meniscal lesions of the knee: a meta-analysis. *J Fam Pract* 2001; 50: 938–44.

Schulman KA, Seils DM, Timbie JW, et al. A national survey of provisions in clinical trial agreements between medical schools and industry sponsors. *N Engl J Med* 2002; 347: 1335–41.

Schwartz LM, Woloshin S. News media coverage of screening mammography for women in their 40s and tamoxifen for primary prevention of breast cancer. *JAMA* 2002; 287: 3136–42.

Sharp PC, Michielutte R, Freimanis R, et al. Reported pain following mammography screening. *Arch Intern Med* 2003; 163: 833–6.

Sharpe M. The report of the Chief Medical Officer's CFS/ME working group: what does it say and will it help? *Clin Med JRCPL* 2002; 2: 427–9.

Sheetz MJ, King GL. Molecular understanding of hyperglycemia's adverse effects for diabetic complications. *JAMA* 2002; 288: 2579–88.

Shepherd J, Cobbe SM, Ford I, et al. Prevention of coronary heart disease with pravastatin in men with hypercholesterolemia. *N Engl J Med* 1995; 333: 1301–7.

Showalter E. *Hystories.* New York: Columbia University Press, 1996.

Shumaker SA, Legault C, Rapp SR, et al. Estrogen plus progestin and the incidence of dementia and mild cognitive impairment in post-menopausal women. *JAMA* 2003; 289: 2651–62.

Silverstein FE, Faich G, Goldstein JL, et al. Gastrointestinal toxicity with celecoxib vs nonsteroidal anti-inflammatory drugs for osteoarthritis and rheumatoid arthritis. The CLASS Study: a randomized controlled trial. *JAMA* 2000; 284: 1247–55.

Simon GE, VonKorff M, Piccinelli M, Fullerton C, Ormel J. An international study of the relation between somatic symptoms and depression. *N Engl J Med* 1999; 341: 1329–35.

Simon JB. Should all people over the age of 50 have regular fecal occult blood tests? (con); Fletcher R. If it works, why not do it? (pro). *N Engl J Med* 1998; 338: 1151–5.

Sloan RP, Bagiella E, VandeCreek L, et al. Should physicians prescribe religious activities? *N Engl J Med* 2000; 342: 1913–6.

Smidt N, van der Windt DA, Assendelft WJ, et al. Corticosteroid injections, physiotherapy or wait-and-see policy for lateral epicondylitis: a randomized controlled trial. *Lancet* 2002; 359: 657–62.

Smith BL. Approaches to breast-cancer staging. *N Engl J Med* 2000; 342: 580–1.

Solomon CG, Dluhy RG. Rethinking postmenopausal hormone therapy. *N Engl J Med* 2003; 348: 579–80.

Sonnenberg A, Delcò F, Inadomi JM. Cost-effectiveness of colonoscopy in screening for colorectal cancer. *Ann Intern Med* 2000; 133: 547–9.

Sox H. Practice guidelines: 1994. *Am J Med* 1994; 97: 205–7.

Sox H. Screening mammography for younger women: back to basics. *Ann Intern Med* 2002; 137: 361–2.

Spiegel BMR, Targownik L, Dulai GS, Garlnek IM. The cost-effectiveness of cyclooxygenase-2 selective inhibitors in the management of chronic arthritis. *Ann Intern Med* 2003; 138: 795–806.

Spitzer WO, LeBlanc F, Dupuis M, et al. Scientific approach to the assessment and management of activity-related spinal disorders. *Spine* 1987; 12 (7S): S1–S59.

Stadtmauer EA, O'Neill A, Goldstein LJ, et al. Conventional-dose chemotherapy compared with high-dose chemotherapy plus autologous hematopoietic stem-cell transplantation for metastatic breast cancer. *N Engl J Med* 2000; 342: 1069–76.

Starr P. *The Social Transformation of American Medicine*. New York: Basic Books, 1982: 96–109.

Steineck G, Helgesen F, Adolfsson J, et al. Quality of life after radical prostatectomy or watchful waiting. *N Engl J Med* 2002; 347: 790–6.

Stelfax HT, Chua G, O'Rourke K, Detsky AS. Conflict of interest in the debate over calcium channel antagonists. *N Engl J Med* 1998; 338: 101–6.

Stone J, Wojcik W, Durrance D, et al. What should we say to patients with symptoms unexplained by disease? the "number needed to offend." *BMJ* 2002; 325: 1449–50.

Strand V, Hochberg MC. The risk of cardiovascular thrombotic events with selective cyclooxygenase-2 inhibitors. *Arthritis Rheum* 2002; 47: 349–55.

Stratton IM, Adler AI, Neil AW, et al. Association of glycaemia with macrovascular and microvascular complications of type 2 diabetes (UKPDS 35): prospective observational study. *BMJ* 2000; 321: 405–12.

Straus SE. Herbal medicines – what's in the bottle? *N Engl J Med* 2002; 347: 1997–8.

Sullivan PF, Smith W, Buchwald D. Latent class analysis of symptoms associated with chronic fatigue syndrome and fibromyalgia. *Psychol Med* 2002; 32: 881–8.

Sutkowski PA, Kannel WB, D'Agostino RB. Changes in risk factors and the decline in mortality from cardiovascular disease. *N Engl J Med* 1990; 322: 1635–41.

Szapary PO, Wolfe ML, Bloedon LT, et al. Guggulipid for the treatment of hypercholesterolemia. *JAMA* 2003; 290: 765–72.

Temple R. Are surrogate markers adequate to assess cardiovascular disease drugs? *JAMA* 1999; 282: 790–5.

Thompson IM, Goodman PF, Tangen CM, et al. The influence of finasteride on the development of prostate cancer. *N Engl J Med* 2003; 349: 215–24.

Thompson PD, Clarkson P, Karas RH. Statin-associated myopathy. *JAMA* 2003; 289: 1681–90.

Thornton H, Dixon-Woods M. Prostate specific antigen testing for prostate cancer. *BMJ* 2002; 325: 725–6.

Thurfjell E. Breast density and the risk of breast cancer. *N Engl J Med* 2002; 347: 866.

Tice JA, Ettinger B, Ensrud K, Wallace R, Blackwell T, Cummings SR. Phytoestrogen supplements for the treatment of hot flashes: the isoflavone clover extract (ICE) study. *JAMA* 2003; 290: 207–14.

Towler B, Irwig L, Glasziou P, et al. A systematic review of the effects of screening for colorectal cancer using the faecal occult blood test, Hemoccult. *BMJ* 1998; 317: 559–65.

Trichopoulou A, Costacou T, Bamia C, Trichopoulos D. Adherence to a Mediterranean diet and survival in a Greek population. *N Engl J Med* 2003; 348: 2599–608.

Trivedi DP, Doll R, Khaw KT. Effect of four monthly oral vitamin D_3 (cholecalciferol) supplementation on fractures and mortality in men and women living in the community: randomized double blind controlled trial. *BMJ* 2003; 326: 455–69.

Tuomilehto J, Lindström J, Eriksson JG, et al. Prevention of type 2 diabetes mellitus by changes in lifestyle among subjects with impaired glucose tolerance. *N Engl J Med* 2001; 344: 1343–50.

Tuomilehto J, Rastenyte D, Birkenhäger WH, et al. Effects of calcium-channel blockade in older patients with diabetes and systolic hypertension. *N Engl J Med* 1999; 340: 677–84.

Turk D. Clinical effectiveness and cost-effectiveness of treatments for patients with chronic pain. *Clin J Pain* 2002; 18: 355–65.

Turner RB. Echinacea for the common cold: can alternative medicine be evidence-based medicine? *Ann Intern Med* 2002; 137: 1001–2.

UKCCCR DCIS Working Party. Radiotherapy and tamoxifen in women with completely excised ductal carcinoma in situ of the breast in the UK, Australia, and New Zealand: randomized controlled trial. *Lancet* 2003; 362: 95–102.

UK Prospective Diabetes Study Group. Intensive blood-glucose control with sulphonylureas or insulin compared with conventional treatment and risk of complications in patients with type 2 diabetes (UKPDS33). *Lancet* 1998; 352: 837–53.

UK Prospective Diabetes Study Group. Tight blood pressure control and risk of macrovascular and microvascular complications in type 2 diabetes (UKPDS 38). *BMJ* 1998; 317: 703–13.

University Group Diabetes Program (UGDP). A study of the effects of hypoglycemic agents on vascular complications in patients with adult-onset diabetes. *Diabetes* 1976; 25: 1129–53.

Urwin M, Symmons D, Allison T, et al. Estimating the burden of musculoskeletal disorders in the community: the comparative prevalence of symptoms at different anatomical sites, and the relation to social deprivation. *Ann Rheum Dis* 1998; 57: 649–55.

US Preventive Services Task Force. Postmenopausal hormone replacement therapy for primary prevention of chronic conditions: recommendations and rationale. *Ann Intern Med* 2002; 137: 834–9.

US Preventive Services Task Force. Screening for breast cancer: recommendations and rationale. *Ann Intern Med* 2002; 137: 344–6.

US Preventive Services Task Force. Screening for colorectal cancer: recommendation and rationale. *Ann Intern Med* 2002; 137: 129–41.

US Preventive Services Task Force. Screening for osteoporosis in postmenopausal women: recommendations and rationale. *Ann Intern Med* 2002; 137: 526–8.

US Preventive Services Task Force. Routine vitamin supplementation to prevent cancer and cardiovascular disease: recommendations and rationale. *Ann Intern Med* 2003; 139: 51–55.

Vahtera J, Kivimäkl M, Pentti J. Effect of organisational downsizing on health of employees. *Lancet* 1997; 350: 1124–8.

Vandenbroucke JP, de Craen AJM. Alternative medicine: a "mirror image" for scientific reasoning in conventional medicine. *Ann Intern Med* 2001; 135: 507–13.

Van Tulder MW, Cherkin DC, Berman B, et al. The effectiveness of acupuncture in the management of acute and chronic low back pain: a systematic review within the framework of the Cochrane Collaboration Back Review Group. *Spine* 1999; 24: 1113–23.

Van Tulder MW, Koes BW, Bouter LM. Conservative treatment of acute and chronic low back pain: a systematic review of randomized controlled trials of the most common interventions. *Spine* 1997; 22: 2128–56.

Van Tulder MW, Malmivaara A, Esmail R, Koes B. Exercise therapy for low back pain. *Spine* 2000; 25: 2784–96.

Van Tulder MW, Scholten RJPM, Koes BW, Deyo RA. Nonsteroidal anti-inflammatory drugs for low back pain. *Spine* 2000; 25: 2501–13.

Varnauskas E and the European Coronary Surgery Study Group. Twelve-year follow-up of survival in the randomized European coronary surgery study. *N Engl J Med* 1988; 319: 332–7.

Vastag B. Study concludes that moderate PSA levels are unrelated to prostate cancer outcomes. *JAMA* 2002; 287: 969–70.

Vercoulen JHMM, Swanink CMA, Fennis JFM, et al. Prognosis in chronic fatigue syndrome: a prospective study on the natural course. *Journal of Neurology, Neurosurgery and Psychiatry* 1996; 60: 489–494.

Verghese J, Lipton RB, Katz MJ, et al. Leisure activities and the risk of dementia in the elderly. *JAMA* 2003; 348: 2508–16.

Veronesi U, Cascinelli N, Mariani L, et al. Twenty-year follow-up of a randomized study comparing breast-conserving surgery with radical mastectomy for early breast cancer. *N Engl J Med* 2002; 347: 1227–32.

Veterans Administration Coronary Artery Bypass Surgery Cooperative Study Group. Eleven-year survival in the Veterans Administration randomized trial of coronary bypass surgery for stable angina. *N Engl J Med* 1984; 311: 1333–9.

Vickers AJ, Fisher P, Smith C, et al. Homoeopathy for delayed onset muscle soreness: a randomized double blind placebo controlled trial. *Br J Sports Med* 1997; 31: 304–7.

Wallace RB. Bone health in nursing home residents. *JAMA* 2000; 284: 1018–9.

Walsh JME, Terdiman JP. Colorectal cancer screening. *JAMA* 2003; 289: 1288–96.

Walsh PC. Surgery and the reduction of mortality from prostate cancer. *N Engl J Med* 2002; 347: 839–40.

Wardwell WI. Chiropractors: evolution to acceptance. In: Gevitz N, ed. *Other Healers: Unorthodox Medicine in America*. Baltimore: Johns Hopkins University Press, 1988: 157–91.

Wassertheil-Smoller S, Hendrix SL, Limacher M, et al. Effect of estrogen plus progestin on stroke in postmenopausal women. *JAMA* 2003; 289: 2673–84.

Wazana A. Physicians and the pharmaceutical industry: is a gift ever a gift? *JAMA* 2000; 283: 373–80.

Weinsier RL, Krumdieck CL. Dairy foods and bone health: examination of the evidence. *Am J Clin Nutrition* 2000; 72: 681–9.

Whelton PK, Appel LJ, Espeland MA, et al. Sodium reduction and weight loss in the treatment of hypertension in older persons. *JAMA* 1998; 279: 839–46.

White KP, Østbye T, Harth M, et al. Perspectives on posttraumatic fibromyalgia: a random survey of Canadian general practitioners, orthopedists, physiatrists, and rheumatologists. *J Rheumatol* 2000; 27: 790–6.

Whiting P, Bagnall AM, Sowden AJ, et al. Interventions for the treatment and management of chronic fatigue syndrome: a systematic review. *JAMA* 2001; 286: 1360–8.

Wilkinson R. *Unhealthy Societies*. London: Routledge, 1996.

Willett WC, Stampfer MJ, Manson JE, et al. Coffee consumption and coronary heart disease in women: a ten-year follow-up. *JAMA* 1996; 275: 458–62.

Williams DA, Cary MA, Groner KH, et al. Improving physical functional status in patients with fibromyalgia: a brief cognitive behavioral intervention. *J Rheumatol* 2002; 29: 1280–6.

Wilson A, Hickie I, Lloyd A, et al. Longitudinal study of outcome of chronic fatigue syndrome. *BMJ* 1994; 308: 756–9.

Wilt TJ, Ishani A, Stark G, et al. Saw palmetto extracts for treatment of benign prostatic hyperplasia: a systematic review. *JAMA* 1998; 280: 1604–9.

Wolfe SM. Direct-to-consumer advertising – education or emotion promotion? *N Engl J Med* 2002; 346: 524–6.

Wolk A, Manson JE, Stampfer MJ, et al. Long-term intake of dietary fiber and decreased risk of coronary heart disease among women. *JAMA* 1999; 281: 1998–2004.

Wolsko PM, Eisenberg DM, Davis RB, et al. Patterns and perceptions of care for treatment of back and neck pain. *Spine* 2003; 28: 292–8.

Woodson G. Dual x-ray absorptiometry T-score concordance and discordance between the hip and spine measurement sites. *J Clin Densitometry* 2000; 3: 319–24.

Woolf SH, Lawrence RS. Preserving scientific debate and patient choice: lessons for the consensus panel on mammography screening. *JAMA* 1997; 278: 2105–8.

Woolhandler S, Campbell T, Himmelstein DU. Costs of health care administration in the United States and Canada. *N Engl J Med* 2003; 349: 768–75.

Writing Group for the Women's Health Initiative Investigators. Risks and benefits of estrogen plus progestin in healthy postmenopausal women. *JAMA* 2002; 288: 321–3.

Index